# Eat Away Illness

# Other Books by the Author

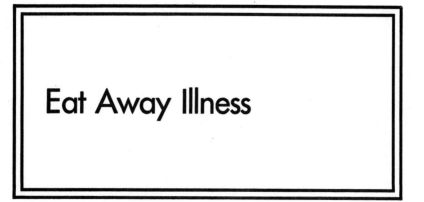

# Eat Away Illness

## How to Age-Proof Your Body With Antioxidant Foods

### Carlson Wade

Parker Publishing Company      West Nyack, New York

This book is a reference work based on research by the author. The opinions expressed herein are not necessarily those of or endorsed by the publisher. The directions stated in this book are in no way to be considered as a substitute for consultation with a duly licensed doctor.

10   9   8   7

Library of Congress Cataloging-in-Publication Data

Wade, Carlson.
    Eat away illness.

    Includes index.
    1. Nutrition.   2. Longevity—Nutritional aspects.
3. Aging—Prevention.   4. Antioxidants—Therapeutic
use.   5. Health.   I. Title.
RA784.W24   1986       613.2′6        85-12367

ISBN 0-13-222613-8

# DEDICATION

To Your New Youth
and Healthy Years Ahead

# Foreword by a Medical Doctor

What can be done to slow the aging process and extend life? These questions have been around as long have human beings themselves. Happily, Carlson Wade provides the answers in this dynamic and powerful book on how to use the newly discovered antioxidants to help defuse "free radicals," the cause of so many illnesses and the aging process itself.

This highly acclaimed medical reporter has devoted years of exhaustive research, spent countless hours interviewing specialists in preventive medicine, and consulted with leading physicians and scientists to come up with a lifesaving book on living a longer and healthier life.

Carlson Wade's book is not just a new theory or a group of special ideas. It is a scientific blending of tested discoveries and proven methods—blended into a miraculous program that really works!

This new book is one that you will read and refer to time and again for the knowledge and helpful programs it offers. From the very first day that you put these methods into use, you will see the glow of youth return to your body and the power of mental energy sweep through your mind. Within a short time, the all-natural antioxidant progress described in this book will help wash out the harmful "free radicals" from your system and put you on the road to a longer and healthier life.

Carlson Wade's book is a major breakthrough in the search for the cause and correction of aging. He has zeroed in on a major cause of illness, namely the presence of "free radical" or harmful substances that bounce around inside body cells. They often damage the cell membranes and the vital nutrients and genetic codes within them. How does one protect against the assault of these inner pollutants, the "free radicals"? How does one wipe them out of the body and therefore build immunity to aging?

Carlson Wade's book tells just how you can provide antioxidants to block much of this "free radical" damage. Available in foods and through various all-natural home programs, these antioxidants are able to combat "free radicals" and defuse their destructive threats. Once you build inner strength through invigorating the cells of the immune system, you are able to insulate yourself against invading organisms that threaten your body with attack.

This amazing discovery of putting antioxidants to work in rebuilding youth from within is one of the most exciting scientific breakthroughs of this era.

Carlson Wade, a leading medical reporter, offers hope for the healing of such problems as aging skin, arthritis, allergies, arteriosclerosis, high blood pressure, overweight, osteoporosis, stress-tension-depression, fatigue, insomnia, low blood sugar, glandular disorder, tight or gnarled muscles, high cholesterol, and much, much more. His book has youth-giving advice for everyone.

Get ready to add healthy, carefree years to your life. You can enjoy the best that is to come with the help of this astonishing and totally commendable book.

Carlson Wade has unlocked the medical secrets that offer you all-natural at-home programs to help you extend your life. More than that, to extend it . . . *youthfully*!

*H. W. Holderby, M.D.*

# What This Book Will Do for You

Are you concerned about the youthfulness of your skin? Do you want to enjoy athletic flexibility of your joints and muscles in your later years? Will you have an alert mind with full memory recall, no matter what your age?

You can extend your prime of life and add many extra years to your life span with the use of a new long-life and "forever young" molecular plan that is based upon the most exciting medical advances to come out of scientific research in years.

It is a totally all-natural approach that uses antioxidants found in everyday foods and beverages that help free your body of pain and discomfort, banish aches and miseries, and wipe away gloom and worry that may be troubling you now.

This book opens the doors of medical and scientific laboratories throughout the world to reveal step-by-step programs using these miracle rejuvenating antioxidants that can give you 10, 20, or more extra years of healthy, carefree, youthful, happy living.

Based on more than a decade of intensive journalistic research, this book draws from the findings of nutritionists, scientists, physicians, biochemists, laboratory technicians, and others in the anti-aging branch of medicine from all corners of the world. Written in easy-to-understand language, it explains the particular health problem that could threaten your youthfulness, and then provides a simple step-by-step program that can help reverse the aging process. Often, results are seen within a very short time!

This book was written as an alternative to the use of harsh drug therapy with its high risk of life-threatening side effects. Instead, it is a unique book because all of the programs and antioxidant remedies are based on completely natural items. Many of the products are probably in your pantry right now, or they are easily available for a modest cost at your local food market. They are specifc anti-aging foods that have been shown in many tests to have rejuvenating and healing properties, which can extend the prime of life from within the body.

With the use of these antioxidant foods, as they are called, you will be able to counteract the wear and tear that may have made you concerned about so-called premature aging. Simply by applying this antioxidant system to your daily life, you will discover a new feeling of health and vitality almost from the start. You will see that you, and only you, are responsible for your new youth. The road to an extended lifeline is in your hands.

This book will show you how to rejuvenate your DNA, genes, and internal aging clock. You will learn how to strengthen your immune system so it becomes a fortress against infection and illness. You are given simple home programs that use antioxidants to rebuild your glandular system so you radiate youthful vitality in body and mind. This book unlocks the mystery of "free radicals" and tells you how you can defuse this major threat to your health.

Because so many youth-seekers have had adverse reactions with drugs, chemicals, surgery, and experimental medications, this book was written to offer a totally natural approach to the goal of total body rejuvenation. No drugs. No medications. No chemicals. No potentially dangerous side effects. Instead, it offers a variety of all-natural foods and products that are harmonious with your natural body. The book is a distillation of hundreds upon hundreds of medical discoveries thoughout the world that have used these all-natural antioxidant programs to restore youth and health to thousands of people. It is easy to understand. It is easy to follow. It is speedy in its rejuvenating results.

Wouldn't you like to wake up each morning bubbling with vitality, eager to enjoy youthful life to the fullest? Of course you would. This book will not only show you how to avoid the dangerous pitfalls of a harmful lifestyle, but also how you can make important changes easily and effectively.

Reading and then using the youth-restoring discoveries in this book is the first step—and it could very well be the most important step you take in your life! And that is just the beginning!

*Carlson Wade*

# Contents

## 3  Free Yourself from Arthritis with the "No-Oxidant" Health Program    26

## 4  How Antioxidants Help You Breathe Easily Without Allergies    38

## 5  How Antioxidants Build Immunity to Arteriosclerosis    50

# The Fountain of Youth Within Your Molecules

1

"May you live a long and healthy life," is the popular toast. But *how* long and *how* healthy is the issue at hand. You want to enjoy an extended life span, but it should be in the prime of life, with the look and feel of total youth. This can be possible with new knowledge that promises to break the aging barrier and extend life—youthfully healthy life—to unlimited horizons. It can be done by getting to the root cause of so-called aging, namely the disintegration of your molecules.

## AGING: WHAT IT IS
## . . .HOW TO REVERSE IT

Regardless of your chronological age, it's a fact of life that you are among the aging. We all are. Aging is a process that commences when we are born. But, until we reach the middle twenties or thirties, the aging process is a positive function; the body grows and develops until it reaches a peak level of size and strength.

**Growing Older Is Slow Process.** From your early thirties onward, the 60 trillion molecules and cells in your bodies start to change. Basically, each cell has a limited life after which it self-reproduces through a process known as *mitosis* or "doubling." The cell dies. While you are reading this page, thousands of your cells are dying. But at the same time many thousands more are being reborn, some faster than others.

*Example:* Fat cells reproduce slowly. Skin cells reproduce about every eight hours. You're also losing about 1,000 brain cells a day that must be replaced if you want to maintain good mental health.

1

From the thirties on, you may think it is all downhill. You may feel it when you see developing wrinkles, find it difficult to keep physically active, and have a negative outlook on things. Check for these signs of so-called aging:

- By age 55 you have a reduced sense of taste.
- You have lost much of your ability to smell.
- Your muscles lack tone, especially facial and arm muscles.
- Hair and nails are easily broken and lack luster.
- Skin looks dry and loses its elasticity, giving you a wrinkled, creased, or sagging appearance.
- An increase in blood pressure. Your arteries become plugged. Your breathing requires more effort. You become easily fatigued.

**Can This "Aging" Be Halted or Reversed?** The answer is that if you use available nutritional and fitness programs, you can call a halt to the "biological clock" that is ticking away your years. You can reconstitute your cells, guard against their early disintegration, rejuvenate your molecules, and tap the "fountain of youth" within your own body. You can do more than refresh your cells, you can rejuvenate your entire body . . . inside and outside!

## SIX CAUSES OF AGING
## —AND HOW TO REVERSE THEM

Longevity scientists and *gerontologists* (specialists in the study of aging) have found that while aging is a complex procedure occurring simultaneously at many levels in the body, it can be categorized under six headings. When you know the reasons why you are aging, you may then use the natural antidotes to reverse the threat to your youth. Check this set of age-causing factors and then set out to use the natural ways to build immunity to these risks.

*1. DNA Damage.* DNA (deoxyribonucleic acid) is the genetic material of nearly all living organisms and is located in your cell nucleus. DNA is a nucleic acid composed of units called nucleotides. The DNA molecule is constantly being damaged by forces within cells and exposure to chemicals that you breathe and eat. Luckily, DNA is biologically empowered with a built-in repair mechanism, but if this is thwarted, aging then takes place as your damaged molecules disintegrate and die. *Youth Remedy:* Protect your DNA by avoiding the use of chemicals as much as possible. Foods and beverages should be as free of additives, preservatives, and artificial flavorings as possible. Read labels. Use fresh foods as much as possible. Protect yourself against environmental pollution. If at all possible, plan to live and work in a healthier and chemical-free atmosphere.

2. *Gene Expression.* Scientists believe that aging can be traced to changes in the activation of specific genes. In brief, a *gene* is the basic unit of genetic material which is carried at a particular place on a chromosome. When the process of gene expression goes awry, the aging clock ticks faster. *Youth Remedy:* Genes depend upon a balance of *amino acids* (the building blocks of protein) to provide nourishment and healthy activation. Provide your genes with amino acids, preferably from a low animal fat source; try combinations of grains, seeds, nuts, legumes, vegetables, and fruits to give youth-extending amino acids to your genes.

3. *Your "Internal" Clock.* The so-called aging signals are supposedly biologically programmed so that your cells die after they have divided a specific number of times. The goal here is to "reset" this "internal" clock so it can be slowed down, perhaps halted. This would slow down the splitting and dying of your cells. *Youth Remedy:* Cells appear to react in a negative manner when assaulted by corrosive substances such as sugar, salt, and caffeine. These substances tend to cause cellular disintegration, even in small amounts. They are believed to "rust" your "internal" clock and cause cellular confusion and the onset of aging. Your simple but lifesaving remedy is to spare your cells the destructiveness of these dangerous poisons. Avoid sugar, salt, and caffeine in all forms and you may well lubricate and control your "internal" clock to work in your favor, not against it!

4. *Your Immune System.* Your body needs the ability to resist infection. Without this inner strength there is a breakdown in immunity and you become vulnerable to one illness after another. Your resistance to infection and aging depends upon a strong and well-nourished immune system. Infants and young people are biologically programmed with strong cells to enable them to resist debilitating illnesses; even if infected, they can recover rapidly because of this inner reserve and strength. Not so with older folks. *Youth Remedy:* Strengthen your store

of lymphocytes or white blood cells, which work together with enzymes to fight off the threat of viral infections. Boost your intake of fresh raw citrus fruits and juices. These are prime sources of bioflavonoids and ascorbic acid, nutrients that replenish your cells and give them power to build your immunity. Oranges, grapefruit, and tangerines and their freshly prepared juices give you this source of immune-building resistance to infection.

5. *Your Brain.* Like other body cells, those of the brain tend to age rapidly. The difference is that unlike other cells (as in the kidney or liver, for instance), brain cells are not replaced as much or as quickly as needed. This means that as you age, you have brain cell loss! Senility, whether simple forgetfulness or complete loss of memory, can be a decisive blow to your health. And it can happen as early as your middle fifties! *Youth Remedy:* Scientists theorize that a nutrient called *choline* is able to strengthen the neurotransmitters or "telegraph signals" between nerve systems in your brain. Choline helps replenish and rejuvenate cells to help you think young. Choline is available as a supplement and is especially potent in a substance called *lecithin.* Derived from soybeans or sunflower seeds, lecithin may well be the key to having a "young mind" in a "young body."

6. *Your Thymus Gland.* Located at the base of your neck, above and in front of your heart, the thymus gland releases hormones that create age-fighting *lymphocytes,* which are white blood cells that produce antibodies to fight off infectious bacteria and oft-killing diseases. A problem here is that after puberty, the thymus gradually shrinks. This means there is a reduction in the hormone *thymosin* as well as cofactors that are supposed to guard you against debilitating illnesses. You may well start to age shortly after puberty! *Youth Remedy:* To help your thymus take up the slack, nourish it with gland-stimulating amino acids from a meatless source, since excessive fat could clog the wheels of this youth clock. Whole grains, pasta, nuts, seeds, legumes, and peas are some of the foods to be included in your diet every day to help your thymus continue releasing the eseential thymosin which is needed to protect you against infections and illnesses. It builds your immunity and that could very well be the most valuable process in your program to extend your prime of life!

When you use these natural methods on a daily basis you will help halt and reverse the aging process so that you will be the picture of youth . . . thanks to healthy molecules and cells—the foundation of rejuvenation.

## Grows Younger in Three Weeks with Six-Step Plan

As a credit manager in a large department store, Marion J. felt energy and youthfulness slipping through her fingers. Although hardly in her middle fifties, she looked twenty years older! Her face had deep creases. Her hair was stringy. She had a stooped posture. Her memory became fuzzy and this was a threat to her responsible position. Marion J. felt a stiffening of her fingers and joints. She caught one allergy after another. Recovery meant a costly confinement and a risk to her job security. She felt displaced by younger people in the office.

She followed a program outlined by a local holistic health practitioner. It called for a six-step improvement in her lifestyle. It was amazingly simple. There was nothing complicated about it. Marion J. was told to eat fresh foods and drink fresh beverages; she was to take nothing processed. She was told to boost her intake of whole grains to provide amino acids *without* the accompanying animal fat. She could have absolutely no sugar, salt, or caffeine in any form. She was to drink more citrus fruits and juices (fresh, not processed) to use lecithin as a daily supplement. Available, in granulated form, lecithin can be sprinkled over a salad or cereal each day.

Within three weeks on this simple six-step plan, which did not call for any drastic changes in her lifestyle, Marion J. was astonished at how it worked. Her face smoothed out. Her hair was thick and youthful. Her posture was erect. Her memory was sharp. She had greater flexibility in her limbs and was remarkably immune to virus infections. She had become amazingly young again. When co-workers asked about her ""secret," she would just say, "I've got young cells." And indeed, the simple six-step plan, based on the preceding six causes of aging and their reversal, had rejuvenated her cells and molecules!

# "FREE RADICALS"— HOW TO DEFUSE THE AGING THREAT

Why we grow old is a problem that has long been pursued by molecular biologists. It appears to be solved by identifying the existence of "free radicals" in the body. These are considered the villains that bring on aging. Defuse these "free radicals" and you may slow or reverse aging and the illnesses of so-called older age.

**What Are Free Radicals?** They are highly reactive molecules produced by low levels of radiation. They are also products of the normal metabolism of fats in our bodies and can result from exposure to chemical toxins as well. Free radicals are damaging to molecules, because each free radical contains an unpaired electron. They can and do attach to other molecules, damaging DNA, cell membranes, and other cell structures.

**How Cellular Destruction Is Caused.** You cannot live without oxygen; it gives you life. But it can also cause destruction. Free radicals, which are tiny molecular fragments, are extremely unstable substances. They are activated by oxygen to combine with unsaturated fats to form peroxides, which damage cells and the protective membrane linings that surround cells. This damage accumulates over the years with tell-tale age spots, wrinkling, and many other worse symptoms.

**You Can See This Process at Work.** Look at a stick of butter that has been left out in the open for a period of time. Look at any other highly perishable foods that are exposed to the elements. They become rancid because of free radical reactions. This happens within your system to your own molecules.

## ANTIOXIDANTS CAN RESCUE YOUR THREATENED CELLS

Your goal is to control the biological process called *oxidation,* which turns fats or lipids into substances that can damage your cells. You need antioxidants as a natural antidote to the threatening power of free radicals.

**What Are Antioxidants?** They are substances that knock out the destructive free radicals. In brief, free radicals contribute to the aging process by damaging your cells. Antioxidants reduce the number of free radicals so that you have more cellular protection. The period of youth lasts much longer.

When damaged by free radicals, DNA can be speedily repaired with the use of antioxidants. These youth-savers also help replace the lipids damaged in the membranes. Antioxidants act as cleansers or "scavengers" in that they seek out and neutralize free radicals, often before any molecular damage is done. So you can see that antioxidants may well be the "fountain of youth" within your body!

# ANTIOXIDANTS HELP YOUR BODY HELP ITSELF

Because antioxidants play a key role in building immunity, they set off an internal reaction that boosts your body's ability to repel invading disease-causing organisms. These infectious bacteria may otherwise cause aging from within. You need to increase your supply of these valuable youth-extending antioxidants.

**Corrects Internal Biological Breakdown.** Molecular damage which leads to premature aging involves a breakdown in which your body's normal defense mechanism goes haywire. Cells may rupture because of the attack of free radicals. To correct against this internal upheaval, antioxidants not only trap the errant and destructive free radicals, but they also build resistance to their oxidative damage. With an abundance of antioxidants you have greater immunity against these unstable and damaging elements.

# THREE POWERFUL REJUVENATING ANTIOXIDANTS

You can find these powerful antioxidants in everyday foods. They go to work immediately in protecting you against the erosion caused by the damaging free radicals. If you include a variety of foods (or even one or two) of each of these three groups in your daily menu, you will be providing a source of rejuvenation from within. It is comparable to having a "fountain of youth" gushing forth in your system. And these foods are so readily available there is no excuse for not having them in your plan for living longer and healthier.

*1. Beta-Carotene.* A predecessor of vitamin A, this is a powerful antioxidant. It is a form of vitamin A that exists in foods of plant origin. Beta-carotene is a very effective quencher of *singlet oxygen,* or toxic substances. It actually devours the damaging free radicals and helps wash them out of your system. *Food Sources:* papaya, sweet potato, collard greens, carrots, cantaloupe, broccoli, butternut squash, watermelon, peaches.

*2. Ascorbic Acid.* You know it as vitamin C. It is needed to repair the molecular damage of *somatic mutations;* that is, errors that alter your cells so they can no longer function properly. This condition not only causes internal breakdown, but leads to aging through the formation of free radicals. Ascorbic acid uses *collagen,* a repair substance, to knit and bind your cells together and guard against free radical formation. Ascorbic acid helps prevent oxidation of many fatty foods, making it an essential antioxidant. *Food Sources:* citrus fruits and their juices, orange, grapefruit, lemon, strawberries, tangerine, guava, green peppers, kale, broccoli, Brussels sprouts, cauliflower, cabbage, tomato, potato.

3. *Selenium.* A little-known but powerful age-fighting trace mineral. It has been reported that in areas of the country with naturally high soil levels of this mineral, there are significantly lower cancer death rates. In contrast, where there is a soil deficiency of selenium, there are higher incidences of cancer of the esophagus, stomach, intestine, rectum, liver, pancreas, larynx, lungs, bladder and the oft-fatal breast malignancy. This antioxidant helps cells live longer by preserving the membrane. Seleniums let various metabolites form into clusters but with an unusual distinction—it lets harmful wastes escape. If the wastes, such as the free radicals, were allowed to remain, then the trillions of cells would die all the sooner. Selenium is a valuable antioxidant that can save your life . . .and save your youth, too. *Food Sources:* whole grains, brans and germs of cereals, broccoli, onions, tomatoes, and tuna. For super antioxidation use selenium *with* vitamin E. This combination builds your immune mechanism for greater protection.

So here are three antioxidants found in everyday foods, which can give you a feeling of total youth in body and mind through their immune-building factors.

## "You Made Me Look Too Young!"

Arthur B. just sat around in an aged slump, even though only in his middle forties. He caught colds easily; his arms and legs felt stiff and creaky. His skin began to wrinkle. He had so much recurring indigestion, he could scarcely eat a balanced diet. With a pasty pallor and a raspy voice, he began to look double his age. Fearing he could be hospitalized, he was soon under the care of a medical nutritionist who diagnosed his problem as a deficiency in antioxidants. Arthur B. was being aged by destructive free radicals.

The medical nutritionist outlined a very simple antioxidant program to help him. Each day, Arthur B. was to include a selection of foods from the beta-carotene, ascorbic acid, and selenium groups. That was the basic program but he also needed to cut down on artificial seasonings such as sugar, salt, chemical additives, and to boost his intake of fresh foods. Results? Within nine days he could move his limbs with youthful agility. His indigestion problem was cured. His skin not only smoothed out, but had a youthful glow that made him look like an athlete. He no longer had respiratory problems. The antioxidant foods had helped him to the point where he quipped to the medical nutritionist, "You made me look too young!" The reply? "The antioxidants restored your youth!"

## 12 STEPS TO HELP YOU LIVE TO BE 100 . . .OR MORE

Set your goal! You want to live to be 100. But you also want to enjoy good health of body and mind as you approach the century mark. You can achieve your goal if you protect yourself against free radicals and build your inner reserves of antioxidants. You can build this inner immunity with the use of a set of steps compiled from findings of longevity scientists, gerontologists, and physicians involved in youth extension.

**Young Cells=Young Body.** This 12-step program will help aid in the regeneration and repair of your trillions of cells by stimulating the synthesis of DNA and its co-worker, RNA (ribonucleic acid), which are concerned with the synthesis of amino acids. The antioxidants used in this 12-step plan also exert potent electro-negative charges on the blood platelets and cells, preventing aggregation of them. This partially explains their importance in clearing plaque from the arteries and therefore protecting you against aging.

Because human fibroblast studies have shown that our cells can live up to 150 years or longer in the appropriate environment, it is necessary for you to create that setting. You need to provide antioxidants and nutrients that will help your inner "fountain of youth" rebuild and regenerate your molecules. This 12-step plan creates that environment.

*1. Stop smoking.* It is responsible for causing cell and molecular deaths and incidences of cancer, perhaps more so than any other substance. Free yourself from smoking and others who smoke, too.

*2. Avoid excessive sun.* Overexposure causes cellular disintegration and the high risk of skin cancer. Moderate amounts of sunshine are helpful because it stimulates the manufacture of vitamin D, which is needed to build a strong bone structure and work with calcium to strengthen your system. Be modest in sun exposure.

*3. Stop drinking alcohol.* It can lead to cellular disintegration to an alarming degree. The dissipation caused by drinking can be seen in young people who look and act much older (and sicker) than their years. Alcohol destroys antioxidants and is involved with formation of free radicals. Avoid alcohol! You'll avoid much aging.

*4. Go easy on fats.* Your diet should be low in fats, especially animal fats. These turn rancid in your system and it is this spoilage that gives rise to free radical formation. A high animal fat diet appears to bring greater risk for developing various cancers. Trim away visible fats before cooking; trim them away before eating. You'll protect yourself against rancidity-oxidation and the threat of molecular destruction. It is best to switch to more healthful vegetable oils.

*5. Take more water and fiber.* Help the antioxidants wash out free radicals by drinking six to eight glasses of water a day. At the same time, boost your intake of high-fiber whole grain cereals and products. This helps in quicker elimination of wastes so that *carcinogens* (cancer-causing substances) do not build up in your digestive tract.

*6. Eat more fruits and vegetables.* Eat foods especially rich in beta-carotene, a powerful and natural antioxidant. Also, with vitamin C and related minerals, they help prevent the activation and formation of many free radicals. Enjoy these plant foods and freshly prepared juices on a daily basis.

*7. Avoid chemicalized foods.* Avoid that which has been salt-cured, salt-pickled, smoked, charred, or moldy! Such foods are so chemicalized, they can destroy antioxidants and make you susceptible to dangerous free radicals. The emphasis is on *fresh* foods whenever possible. Bake, broil, steam, or boil, but do not resort to these chemicalized methods that destroy food value and your cells!

*8. Be cautious about x-rays.* Even moderate doses of invasive radiation can destroy valuable cells, sometimes permanently. Always ask if these x-rays are really necessary or are just routine. Be sure your dentist provides a lead-lined apron with a thyroid-protecting collar when giving you any necessary x-rays.

*9. Control your weight.* Obesity breaks down your immune system. It can clog your cells and make you vulnerable to endless ailments. Obesity is a thief of life. Remain within healthy weight levels and you have a good chance of living longer.

*10. Reduce or conrol stress.* It causes the secretion of substances that weaken your immune system, thus decreasing your ability to fight off diseases. Unrelieved or prolonged stress can be a killer via cardiovascular troubles as well as hypertension to name just a few problems. Try to avoid stress!

*11. Fish oils are helpful.* They contain ingredients believed to protect against free radical clumping that could predispose heart attack. Plan to include fish liver oils on a daily basis. Just two tablespoons mixed with a vegetable juice taken daily can boost so many antioxidants that you can rebuild your health in a short while.

*12. Eat more plant foods.* Not only do they have a lower fat content, but their protein stabilizes your blood cholesterol levels. Remember that animal fat rancidity is the cause for formation of free radicals. Don't "eat" free radicals in the form of animal fats! A moderate amount, balanced with more plant foods, will help guard against free radical overload. Plant foods are high in antioxidants to keep your immune system working well to slow the aging process.

When you build this 12-step plan into your daily lifestyle you will see the benefits almost at once: clearer skin; better digestion; more flexible body; youthful alertness. You will look and feel younger, almost from the first few days on this plan.

Of course you want to maximize vigor and vitality in your years. You do want to live to be 100, but with a youthful body and mind. That is your goal, and you can reach it with a quick and lively step when you set your goal on the buildup of antioxidants, the "fountain of youth" within your molecules. You will then fulfill the toast of living a "long and healthy life!"

## HIGHLIGHTS

1. The secret of perpetual youth is in your trillions of cells. Keep them healthy and you have a good chance for a long and youthful life.
2. Check the six basic causes of aging and the youth remedies that work almost from the first day.
3. Marion J. rejuvenated herself in three weeks on this six-step plan.

4. Use antioxidants in everyday foods to defuse free radicals, the real cause of aging.
5. Use the three powerful rejuvenating antioxidants and rescue your cells from premature aging.
6. Arthur B. was aging so rapidly he feared confinement in a hospital. He followed a simple program drawn up by his medical nutritionist that included three special food groups. Within little time, he was totally rejuvenated and quipped that he looked too young!
7. Live to be 100 . . .or more on an easy 12-step plan that improves your lifestyle. It establishes a "fountain of youth" within your molecules. It helps you grow healthier and seem younger as you celebrate more birthdays!

# 2

# How Biological Molecular Foods Can Give You A "Forever Young" Skin At Any Age

Your skin is a barometer of your health. If your cheeks have a rosy glow; if you have that dew-kissed fresh look; if your skin has a silky smoothness that is free from creases or wrinkles, then you have youthful skin.

If you have a sallow or pallid look; if your face is like parchment and wrinkles mar what should be total youthfulness, then your skin has fallen victim to the accumulation of the age-causing and molecule-destroying free radicals. You need to make a number of nutritional corrections to help wash out these destructive elements and rebuild your skin so it can be a mirror of your new health.

## WHY YOUR SKIN AGES —HOW BIOLOGICAL FOODS CAN REJUVENATE IT

An accumulation of these free radicals resulting from oxidative reactions in the body tend to speed up the skin-aging process. If allowed to build up, these wastes initiate the accumulation of an oxidized pigmented lipid called *lipofuscin,* which can be seen in the form of "age spots" and blemishes. Wrinkles and folds appear and you have the problem of aging skin.

To understand how a certain group of foods can erase these accumulative pigments and help you revive and rejuvenate your skin, it is helpful to know the basics about your skin structure.

Your skin is composed of three major layers:

1. Epidermis. The true outer barrier which protects your body. It is composed of dead cells (as are the nails and hair) which are contin-

uously shed and replaced by new cells from the layers below. It normally contains about ten percent water.

2. Dermis. Acts as a support for the epidermis and contains nerves, blood vessels, hair follicles, sweat and sebaceous (skin lubricant) glands as well as supportive cellular tissue.

3. Subcutaneous tissue. Composed mostly of fat cells. It provides flexibility to your skin and padding for underlying tissue.

**Checklist of Aging Signs.** Your skin can start to show signs of aging in your late twenties. The epidermis has flat, dead cells that tend to accumulate. This gives your skin a coarser, duller appearance. Your pores appear larger. As your sweat glands become clogged with dead cells, they lose efficiency and provide less of the needed moisture. Your oil glands also become blocked with these fragments and cannot provide the important lubrication. The problem is that oil is needed to protect against evaporation of natural moisture; without adequate lubrication, more moisture is lost and your skin dries, bringing on the appearance of old age. This condition can happen when you are in your prime of life!

How can you guard against this threat to your skin? How can you uproot and wash out these waste products so that your sweat and oil glands can function freely to give you a dewy fresh skin?

Antioxidant foods are able to search out, gather up, and help eliminate these causes of aging skin. In particular, one group of foods, beta-carotene foods, have this inner-cleansing power to give you a youthful skin. Beta-carotene has been used at exclusive Swiss spas for many years, and the secret was not revealed until just recently. Now you can use this same skin rejuvenation program right at home and see your skin become younger from the first day.

## MILLION-DOLLAR SWISS SPA YOUTH SECRET

At several of these plush youth spas tucked in the mountains of Switzerland, where only the elite society and the "beautiful people" can afford to take the treatment, the secret was to use beta-carotene to clear up the skin, smooth out wrinkles, and restore "blushing youth" to the firm face. Investigative journalism was able to learn the all-natural and amazingly effective secret that transformed crease-lined women into sleek, smooth-faced beauties. And many are in their seventies and eighties!

**Beta Carotene Is the Beauty Secret.** This is a form of vitamin A that exists in foods of plant origin. It is transformed into skin-rejuvenating vitamin A via your intestinal-digestive system. Once this antioxidant nutrient enters your system, it quickly goes to work to get rid of the age-causing free radicals. Here is what happens and why beta-carotene is a million-dollar youth secret:

*Problem:* Respiration, or the reduction of oxygen molecules in your cells, produces oxidative radicals and peroxides which are too reactive to be tolerated. They can cause aging almost overnight. These are free radicals that destroy healthy cells. They attack the collagen that holds such cells together. The bombardment of collagen by these free radicals causes it to become inflexible, a primary factor in the aging process. This may also lead to inflammation of various tissues and a breakdown in the tissue structure so that you have sagging skin.

*Solution:* Beta-carotene is an antioxidant that tends to "mop up" these free radicals and prepare them for elimination. Beta-carotene will enter into the cell membrane and strengthen its ability to fight and survive the constant free radical attacks. It is like having a fortress-like form of biological molecular protection that can keep out harmful invaders.

This is the basis of the rejuvenation program for which many members of top society have all paid unlimited money in order to have younger skin. The program called for the use of beta-carotene foods as part of a general health and fitness program at a plush and scenic Swiss health spa. You need not pay the million-dollar tab to reap the benefits. You can roll back the years by following this same simple skin-rejuvenating program right at home.

## HOW TO USE THESE YOUTH-RESTORING FOODS

Because beta-carotene is transformed into vitamin A, you must take a basic minimum each day. The Recommended Dietary Allowance for adults is 5,000 International Units of vitamin A for men, and 4,000 for women. This is a daily minimum. Plan to (1) use these foods as snacks throughout the day to replace refined sugar and calorie-high confections; (2) include them as part of a vegetable platter with your main meal every day; (3) use several vegetables as a main meal; (4) use the fruit as part of a salad; (5) use some of the fruits for dessert.

*Remember:* The beta-carotene can uproot and dislodge the age-causing free radicals but only if available on a *daily* basis. Just plan your menu to include a variety of these beta-carotene foods and your skin will reward you with a smooth appearance almost overnight, as was seen in the million-dollar health spas of Switzerland.

# 18 BETA-CAROTENE FOODS THAT GIVE YOU "FOREVER YOUNG" SKIN

## Foods Richest in Carotene

| Food | Serving | Carotene (I.U.) |
|---|---|---|
| Papaya | ½ medium | 8,867 |
| Sweet potato | ½ cup, cooked | 8,500 |
| Collard greens | ½ cup, cooked | 7,917 |
| Carrots | ½ cup, cooked | 7,250 |
| Chard | ½ cup, cooked | 6,042 |
| Beet greens | ½ cup, cooked | 6,042 |
| Spinach | ½ cup, cooked | 6,000 |
| Cantaloupe | ¼ medium | 5,667 |
| Broccoli | ½ cup, cooked | 3,229 |
| Squash, butternut | ½ cup, cooked | 1,333 |
| Watermelon | 1 cup | 1,173 |
| Peaches | 1 large | 1,042 |
| Squash, yellow | ½ cup, cooked | 900 |
| Apricots | 1 medium | 892 |
| Squash, hubbard | ½ cup, cooked | 667 |
| Squash, zucchini | ½ cup, cooked | 600 |
| Prunes | ½ cup, cooked | 417 |
| Squash, acorn | ½ cup, cooked | 234 |

**Vitamin A Is a Biological Skin Food.** You may find that vitamin A can have a beneficial reaction, more so than beta-carotene. For some people it can be a biological skin food. It can strengthen and stabilize the cellular membrane system and fortify resistance against damage by the free radicals. You can plan your menu to include these vitamin A foods in your diet.

*Warning:* Vitamin A is found largely in foods of animal origin that are also high in saturated fats and cholesterol. For this reason, such foods are not highly recommended by the Swiss health spas. You may still want to use them in moderation, of course. A small serving of liver, a pat of butter, a soft-boiled egg, for example, will give you goodly amounts of skin-nourishing vitamin A with appreciable levels of the fatty elements. Just aim for a balance between beta-carotene and vitamin A, if that is your choice.

## 10 VITAMIN A FOODS
## THAT HELP CLEAR UP YOUR SKIN

## Foods Richest in Vitamin A

| Foods | Units of vitamin A in one serving (about 3½ ounces) |
|---|---|
| Liver, beef | 53,500 |
| Liver, calf | 32,200 |
| Liver, chicken (1 cup) | 17,200 |
| Liverwurst (½ lb) | 7,200 |
| Eggs, 2 | 1,140 |
| Milk, whole (1 cup) | 350 |
| Cream, half and half (1 cup) | 1,160 |
| Cream, light (1 cup) | 2,020 |
| Butter (1 tsp) | 160 |
| Cheese (1 ounce) | 370 |

### How Beta-Carotene Created
### Overnight Rejuvenation

Helen E. almost wept to see herself in the mirror. Her chin sagged and her cheeks were wrinkled folds. Age spots blemished her face. Large pores gave her an unsightly look. Crease lines appeared whenever she smiled (which was rare!) or moved her mouth. At a loss for what to do, she asked a visiting nurse from abroad what the secret of her smooth skin could be. Both were in their early fifties, but the European nurse looked half her age because of her smooth face and glowing appearance.

The nurse told of the beta-carotene program. All she had to do was to plan to boost intake of these foods on a daily basis. For severe wrinkling and aging problems, she recommended going on a simple beta-carotene "fasting" program. That is, for five days eat little else but beta-carotene foods. She confided that the most hopeless cases of wrinkled and skin-aged women who came to the Swiss health spas responded dramatically to such a program.

Helen E. tried it. She gave up refined foods and enjoyed a variety of beta-carotene foods. She was astonished at how this antioxidant was able to clear up her skin. Within one or two days, her chin firmed up. Her cheeks bloomed like dew-kissed rose petals and became smooth as silk. Age spots just faded away and pores tightened. When she smiled (which was more often now), she looked like a youngster with a crease-free happy face. She was helped within three days. Beta-carotene was to be her "youth food" from now on!

## RESTORE THE PH FACTOR
## AND WATCH YOUR SKIN BECOME YOUNGER

The pH factor refers to your body's acid-alkaline balance. Youthful, healthy skin has an acid mantle to protect it from bacterial invasion. If this acid mantle is disturbed or imbalanced, the skin becomes vulnerable to both external and internal invasion and contamination. This upset in balance happens whenever you wash your face or let your skin become deficient in essential, but easily available, antioxidants.

**What Is Good pH Level?** Actually, pH is a measure of the concentration of hydrogen ions in a solution, and therefore of its acidity or alkalinity. A pH of 7 indicates a neutral solution. A pH below 7 indicates acidity. A pH in excess of 7 indicates alkalinity. *Easy Test:* Ask your pharmacist for nitrazine paper, a good testing device. Follow package instructions on applying to your skin. Your mantle will have a pH range anywhere from 5.2 to 6 within a scale of 4.5 to 7.5 on this paper. Remember, the lower number represents the acid side of the scale; the higher denotes an alkaline state. A measurement of about 5.5 would give you a good balance. This varies according to individuals but it is a basic rule of thumb.

**Are You Washing Away Your Protective Mantle?** To keep your skin looking and feeling its best it must be cleansed gently and moisture-sealed effectively. You may think this can be done with soap. Right? *Wrong!*

Soap is tallow based. It has an alkaline pH that disturbs your skin's outermost protective layer, the "acid mantle." Furthermore, soap can be harsh; it strips away your skin's natural moisture and causes a dryness and tightness that brings on wrinkles. With your pores vulnerable to external pollution, cellular disintegration may occur, which gives rise to the accumulation of floating debris. Free radicals or wastes take hold and break down the protective structure that supports your skin from beneath, which can lead to premature aging. You can readily appreciate the importance of maintaining a proper "acid mantle" to guard against this threat. And you do want to keep your skin clean, so you would do well to select a soap that is pH balanced. Ask your pharmacist or health store for such a soap. Your dermatologist will be able to advise a cleanser for your particular skin type, too. This will help cleanse your skin and protect against upsetting your personal pH level.

## THE FRUIT THAT REJUVENATES YOUR SKIN IN MINUTES

Your skin has something in common with one delicious fruit, the strawberry. *Both have the same pH.* This biological molecular finding can give you a "fresh-as-springtime" skin almost in minutes.

You can use this amazing skin-feeding strawberry to help balance the acid-alkaline level and restore pH to slough off wastes that otherwise are responsible for aging.

**Strawberry Facial.** Ancients would crush the berries, mix them with a bit of water, and apply to areas of your skin in need of rejuvenation. Let the mixture remain on for 30 minutes. Splash off with tepid water. The ascorbic acid and enzymes in the fruit seep through your skin pores, help dissolve some of the wastes, and facilitate in their elimination. Your skin will have a chance to glow from within.

*Suggestion:* A famous New York City skin care center mashes strawberries in equal amounts of water. They prescribe an application before retiring to the aging skin areas. A softening-cleansing-rejuvenation occurs *while you sleep.* The next morning, wash it off and you will be surprised at the smooth skin you see. It glows with the freshness of youth!

## Erases Blemishes, Smooths Wrinkles

Nothing could remove the age lines or unsightly bumps and pimples on the face, neck, and arms of Martha K. As a private secretary to a fashion consultant, she did not create a good impression with her aging skin! She took to wearing clumsy long-sleeved clothes with high collars, and covered her face with garish makeup. Martha K. could hardly look at herself; she felt self-conscious about the stares of others in the world of fashion and beauty in which she mixed.

She happened to meet a visiting dermatologist who was attending a convention. He saw her blemishes and suggested she try this simple home remedy: mash equal amounts of strawberries and water to make a puree or paste. Apply like a cream over blemishes and wrinkles. The next morning, just rinse the cream off. Nothing else. Do this every night until you see the results.

Doubtfully, Martha K. tried the remedy. Since she had gone the route of one patent remedy after another with no clearing up of her skin problems she was naturally dubious. But since it cost almost nothing, and was recommended by a dermatologist, she decided to give it a try.

Just one overnight berry application proved to be nothing short of a miracle. Martha K. could scarcely believe the youthful reflection that stared at her from the mirror the next morning. Her wrinkles were almost gone. There was no trace of bumps or blemishes. Her arms were swan-like in soft smoothness. She had a lovely throat line and felt young again. She looked young! Thanks to a simple home remedy using strawberries, she was no longer ashamed of her skin. She was a glamour girl, so to speak, and it happened overnight!

# THE GOLDEN FRUIT THAT ERASES AGE LINES

The familiar golden lemon may well be the most important youth extender your skin will ever require. It is especially useful because its natural tartness and high supply of ascorbic acid can correct any pH imbalance. It restores a natural acid mantle. The lemon is similar to an antioxidant in that it penetrates your pores, attracts the broken off pieces of molecules that are threatening your skin structure, and aids in their dissolution and removal. This antioxidant fruit should be used on a regular basis to help do more than give you a youthful skin; it will help you maintain a lifetime bloom of youthfulness.

### How to Use the Antioxidant Lemon for Skin Rejuvenation

1. Lemon Facial. Rub half a lemon over your face after washing to restore tissue integrity and pH balance.

2. Young Hands. Squeeze half a lemon into warm water and soak your hands for 15 minutes. Or, rub your hands with a lemon wedge. The antioxidant factors will lighten so-called age pigments; the clusters of molecular fragments will be dissolved and eliminated to give you young hands.

3. Smooth Face. After washing, squeeze and strain a little fresh lemon in your rinse water to help get rid of every trace of soap which may have taken away your protective acid mantle. Rinse over and over with clear water. You'll soon have a golden smooth face.

4. Rough Elbows Become Soft, Smooth. Place your rough elbows into two halves of cut lemons to help get rid of free radicals you can see as dry, scaly skin. The antioxidant factors in the lemons will soften, smooth, and whiten your elbows.

5. Soften Your Feet. The thickest areas of your skin are the soles of your feet (about 0.1 millimeter) and also are the most vulnerable to dryness. Your sebaceous glands often reduce production of oily substances in your feet and therefore an accumulation of molecular wastes can cause hardening of the skin in this area. Just rub a wedge of fresh lemon on the skin of your feet to soften the skin. This helps to refresh sore feet too. Or, soak your feet in a mixture of hot water and the juice of one whole lemon. Rinse in warm water and dry gently. You'll see how the antioxidants in the lemon have helped whiten, soften, soothe your feet almost immediately.

6. Lemon-Oatmeal Facial Mask. Scrub away your metabolic fallout with a twice-a-week facial mask. *Benefit:* It gets rid of the dull,

muddy look, and dirt and excessive oils that are making you look haggard. Here's how to rejuvenate your face in minutes: Mix together the juice of one lemon and the white of one egg. Add dry oatmeal gradually until you have a soft paste. Mix with a slight chopping motion, then allow to set a few minutes till the moisture is absorbed. Apply to your face, avoiding areas around the eyes. Let dry for about ten minutes, then splash off with tepid water. Your wrinkles, crease lines, blemishes, age spots, and sagging areas should be less noticeable. *Reason:* The antioxidants of the lemon combine with the lecithin in the egg white and join with the amino acids of the oatmeal to create a deep pore cleansing. These ingredients uproot the offensive fragments and remove them from your dermis and subcutaneous tissues. Within moments, you have a youthful skin.

7. Facial Refresher. Give your face a pick-me-up on a hot day (or any day). Fill an ice cube tray with equal parts strained lemon juice and water. Freeze. Lightly rub one of the lemon cubes over your face and neck. Rinse with cool water and pat dry. Your face feels as refreshed as if you'd splashed it in a mountain stream.

8. Lemon Water. This is a good item to keep in your refrigerator. Mix it up in any quantity you prefer, using this easy formula: For every cup of strained lemon juice, add half a cup of water. It is handy as a base for mixing all other formulas. Use in facials, for manicures, and so forth. This saves you the effort of squeezing a lemon every time. The mixture keeps well when refrigerated.

9. Overall Skin Rejuvenator. Slice several fresh lemons into your warm bath and step in. The lemon oils release their sun-blessed fragrance all through the bathroom. The freshening lemon juices are antioxidants in that they perk you up all over and keep harmful soap film from clogging your pores. You'll emerge with a totally young-looking body.

10. Scalp-Hair Pickup. Your scalp is skin and the shedding you know as pesky dandruff is the result of the fragments in your dermis and subcutaneous layers. Dandruff is an accumulation of free radicals! These are the wastes you want to get rid of in order to have a clean and healthy scalp and youthful hair. The antioxidants in lemon juice work almost immediately to perform a double benefit: (1) they restore the valuable pH acid-alkaline balance; (2) they wash away and dissolve clogging free radicals known as dandruff flakes that choke hair follicles and could predispose hair loss. *Simple Remedy:* After shampooing, just

cut a fresh lemon in half and squeeze it over your hair. It helps get rid of damaging soap film and excess oiliness. It leaves your hair looking squeaky-clean and smelling lemon-fresh. This is a scalp and hair rejuvenation.

## THE ANTIOXIDANT FOOD CREAM THAT ERASES 10-20-30 YEARS FROM YOUR SKIN . . .WITHIN THREE DAYS OR LESS

A major cause of your so-called aging is the problem of "cross-linkage." That is when free radicals bind together large molecules. These are cross-links that form in the connective tissue that binds cells together. Even DNA itself, within the nucleus of a cell, is vulnerable to the aging reaction of cross-linkage. Neglected, it can accumulate until these large molecular clusters erupt as wrinkled folds, age spots, blemishes. To help uproot and cast out the large molecules or cross-links, the use of antioxidants in a special food cream can work wonders.

**Three Simple Ingredients.** An ordinary cucumber and powdered milk together with egg white can join forces to create an antioxidant reaction that can take years off your skin . . .in a few days.

*How to Prepare:* Blend together one-half cup of sliced cucumber, three teaspoons of ordinary powdered milk, and one egg white. When it becomes a smooth cream or paste, apply with your finger tips in a gentle upward motion all over your face and neck. Use a bit more pressure (gently, please) on those trouble spots. Let mixture remain from 30 to 45 minutes. Splash off with warm and then cool water. Blot dry. Immediately, you can see the fading away of telltale age spots and blemishes.

**The Skin-Saving Benefits of Antioxidant Food Cream.** The valuable minerals of sulfur and silicon in the cucumber blend with the calcium in the milk and become empowered by the protein and lecithin of the egg white. This triple power creates an invigorating antioxidant reaction deep within your skin pores to scour away the damaging cross-links that might otherwise become wrinkled furrows and blemishes. This simple antioxidant skin cream works within days to give you that youthful skin you crave.

### Reverses Aging in Three Days

Troubled because no cosmetics could correct her sagging skin, Anna T. sought the help of a nutritionally oriented cosmetician who explained that she had to cleanse away the accumulated debris with the use of antioxidants.

She gave Anna T. the simple recipe for the antioxidant food cream and suggested she try it once a day. Anna prepared the cream and gently rubbed it into her aging skin. Within two days, she could see the crease lines starting to fade away. The blemishes flattened out. Blotches just disappeared. At the end of the third day, and the third application of this antioxidant food cream, Anna T. remarked that she felt and looked 20 years younger. The cream had uprooted and eliminated the age-causing cross-links and had given her a new lease on the lifeline of youth.

# EVERYDAY FRUIT ERASES "AGE SPOTS" ON HANDS

So-called "age spots" that you see on your hands (and elsewhere) are also called "liver spots" (which is a misnomer, since this organ has nothing to do with the accumulation of free radicals on your hands).

Rather, these brown spots, called *lentigines,* are the result of a change in color pigmentation because of the clusters of cross-links in certain parts of your body. They seem to gather on the backs of your hands, and more than anywhere else, they are more noticeable.

**How Fruit Lightens Spots.** The ordinary pineapple is a concentrated source of an enzyme called *bromelain.* It helps dissolve the layer of dead cells to rid your skin of this dead tissue buildup that can be seen as brown spots. You can apply pineapple juice to these spots and watch them fade away in a short time.

Prepare one-fourth cup of freshly squeezed pineapple juice. (Avoid canned or frozen or processed pineapple juice, because the enzyme is destroyed with this manufacturing method. The juice must be fresh to work.) Soak a double thickness of a clean cloth in the juice. Place this gauze on your skin wherever you see the so-called aging spots. The skin should be free of cream or oil and preferably freshly washed. Let this pineapple-juice-soaked gauze remain for 20 minutes. Then splash off in warm water and pat dry. You should see a layer of skin peel off; this shows that the bromelain enzyme has worked to remove the dead cells. The same enzyme has penetrated to dissolve the lentigines, or cross-links, and will soon clear up your skin.

You may need to use this simple fruit treatment for several applications, but within a few days, you will discover that it has used its antioxidant power via the bromelain enzymes to dissolve and cast out the cross-links from your skin. Your so-called age spots will just fade away.

Your skin is the largest organ of your body. Keep it looking young with biological molecular foods. It will make you feel young, too, no matter what your age, thanks to antioxidants and the use of everyday foods to correct the problem of free radicals.

# IN REVIEW

1. Get acquainted with your skin and alert yourself to aging signs that call for speedy corrective healing.
2. A million-dollar Swiss spa had a secret for speedy rejuvenation with the use of tasty beta-carotene foods. They created overnight rejuvenation for Helen E.
3. Restore the pH factor and give yourself youthful skin.
4. Just one overnight strawberry facial erased blemishes, smoothed wrinkles, and put the bloom of youth into the skin of Martha K.
5. The ordinary lemon has powerful antioxidant factors that can rejuvenate your skin in minutes.
6. Troubled with aging, sagging skin, Anna T. used an antioxidant cream that reversed the threat of wrinkling within three days.
7. Annoying or telltale "age spots" on hands (and elsewhere) can be traced to cross-linkage accumulation. The ordinary pineapple can lighten and eliminate these brown spots.

# 3

# Free Yourself from Arthritis with the "No-Oxidant" Health Program

Living well is possible if you are free of the risk of arthritis. Often called "everybody's illness," it does affect every person in some way, directly or indirectly, physically or economically. Does it have to happen? With the proper use of a "no-oxidant" health program, you can not only build immunity to the problem of arthritis, but you will be able to uproot and cast this crippler out of your system, even if it has been a problem for many years.

## WHAT IS ARTHRITIS?

The word *arthritis* literally means inflammation of a joint. The term is widely used, however, to cover close to 100 different conditions which cause aching and pain in joints and connective tissues throughout the body, not all of them necessarily involving inflammation. There are two most common forms of arthritis:

1. Rheumatoid. This is the most serious because it can lead to crippling. It is inflammatory and often chronic. Although it primarily attacks the joints, it can also cause disease in the lungs, skin, blood vessels, muscles, spleen, and heart. It tends to flare up and subside unpredictably, often causing progressive damage to tissues. Women are affected three times more often than men. In youngsters it occurs in a form know as *juvenile rheumatoid arthritis* and can be quite serious.

2. Osteoarthritis. This is also called degenerative joint disease, which is principally caused by wear-and-tear on the joints and happens with advancing age, often starting in the forties. It is usually mild and

not too inflammatory. Sometimes there can be considerable pain. Mild to severe disability may develop gradually.

## FOUR WARNING SIGNS OF POSSIBLE ARTHRITIS

Aches and pains in and around joints can mean so many different things—dozens of different conditions—so it is essential to get a proper medical diagnosis. If signs or systems appear, *do not delay*; see your doctor. The sooner your holistic health practitioner examines your condition, the better your chances of recovery. Basically, there are four warning signs that should call for speedy medical evaluation:

1. Persistent pain and stiffness when getting up in the morning.
2. Pain, tenderness, or swelling in one or more joints.
3. Recurrence of these symptoms, especially when they involve more than one joint.
4. Recurrent or persistent pain and stiffness in the neck, lower back, knees and other joints.

When you experience either one or more of these warning signs, seek medical testing and diagnosis at once.

## CAUSE: ERROR IN METABOLISM

To strike at the root of arthritis, it is important to consider an underlying cause, namely that of an error in metabolism. Something has gone awry with your system and free-floating bacteria have invaded your joints. This leads to an infection that could cause joint-muscle-tissue inflammation and injury. In order to promote healing, the goal is to correct the cause *first*, and then correct the symptoms *second*.

It is true that there is a wide variety of antibiotics, medications, drugs, and anti-inflammatory products in either prescription or over-the-counter forms. They promise to relieve your symptoms but not correct the cause. And while you will have some respite from pain, you will have to keep taking medication on a permanent basis. They offer *temporary* relief, at best.

A further problem with chemotherapy is that drugs do cause side effects. They could create gastrointestinal disorders, internal bleeding, audio-visual blurring, skin eruptions, or vertigo, to name just a few reactions. Sometimes, the "cure" is worse than the illness!

**Metabolic Error Needs Correction.** To free yourself from arthritis, you need to get to the cause, which can be a metabolic error. There is a destruction of cellular integrity. During metabolism, the chromosome changeover of oxygen to water will produce hydrogen peroxide and hydroxyl radicals. These are mutagenic and biologically destructive—the harmful free radicals that are the byproducts of a disturbed oxidative process. They may be considered metabolic errors which need correction if you expect to get rid of arthritis in any of its forms.

**How Oxidative Radicals Cause Arthritis.** These fragmentary molecules pierce the interior of cartilage and thereby damage their functioning organelles. The cartilage becomes frayed. In an effort to repair itself, the new cartilage formed is not as durable as the original. The adjacent bone grows spurs or overgrowths around the joint. The destructive free radical fragments wear away the cartilage so completely in places that the bone ends themselves grate against each other. You can feel this reaction by stiffness in your joints; occasionally a grating noise can be heard coming from your joint when it is moved. You have a limited range of motion, and after excessive use or injury you will experience pain, swelling, and tenderness of the joint because of inflammation. The free radicals have brought on arthritis.

## SAY GOODBYE TO ARTHRITIS WHEN YOU SAY GOODBYE TO NIGHTSHADE FOODS

In certain biologically programmed individuals, the eating of a group of foods belonging to the *nightshade* family can deposit a toxic waste that can cause a proliferation of the harmful oxidative radicals.

This is similar to an allergic reaction. Arthritis begins and continues because you are eating certain foods that are depositing bone- and cartilage-disintegrating free radicals. To put it briefly, your arthritis may be caused by certain foods.

**What Are Nightshade Foods? What Are Their Dangers?** These are crop plants that may be nutritious to some people but antagonistic to others. The group consists of four basic foods:

white potatoes, eggplant, tomatoes, and green or red peppers. They release a substance called *solanine* that enters your cells, destroys their functions, kills them and deposits wastes that are the familiar free radicals. This triggers the arthritis reaction.

**Solanine Causes Cross-Linkage.** Cross-linkage is a damaging condition in which solanine causes the large molecules to be bound together; cross-linking two molecules is the same as handcuffing two workers on an assembly line; they become handicapped or completely incapacitated. Cross-links will form in the connective tissue that binds cells together and can be responsible for the stiffness-brittleness-inflammation that accompanies arthritis. This all begins when solanine, the toxic substance in the nightshade foods, enters the system.

**Are You Allergic to Solanine?** Each person is as different as fingerprints are from one another. Many are able to enjoy the nightshade foods listed above and enjoy their nutritional benefits, but many others experience a negative reaction to these foods. It may happen all at once or it may worsen over a period of time. If you have found that your joints are stiff, your muscles are losing flexibility, your spine is less moveable, then you may be allergic to solanine from the nightshade family. You need to self-test your responses when you eliminate them in all forms. A health practitioner can guide you in this.

## Avoids Nightshades, Avoids Arthritis in Six Days

Construction foreman Ben A. was on the verge of losing his lucrative position and becoming a disability pensioneer. He had agonizing aches in his upper back; his spine was stiff. He felt wrenching pains when he had to jockey his position on steel girders. Even on the ground he had difficulty moving about. Although in his early fifties and always a vigorous worker, he was about to concede defeat to advancing arthritis.

A sports physician who was aware of the reaction of certain foods on the metabolic system was a neighbor of Ben A. Listening to his problems, he suggested the elimination of these four foods: white potatoes, eggplants, tomatoes, and green or red peppers. No other treatment or program was prescribed. Ben A. was skeptical but so tortured with shooting pain spasms and the risk of being jobless, he followed the simple program.

Within three days the construction foreman was able to do

his arduous construction work with reduced pain and inflammation. At the end of the sixth day, he was overjoyed. He said he was cured of arthritis, thanks to the recommended "no nightshade" program!

## HOW TO FOLLOW THE "NO NIGHTSHADE" DIET AND BUILD IMMUNITY TO ARTHRITIS

Granted, these nightshade vegetables are healthy foods, but to certain people they could trigger off allergic reactions that are identified as arthritis. For these, a "no nightshade" diet plan is a biological way to build immunity to this crippling condition. It can also reverse arthritis, uproot its causes, and cast it out of the system. Even those with advanced cases of arthritis will find it helpful, perhaps healing, to be on the program. But it calls for a bit of planning.

**Always Read Labels.** Whenever you consider a packaged food, read the list of ingredients. If any of the four foods are included, it is best to pass it by.

**Use Fresh Foods.** To avoid the risk of consuming hidden nightshade ingredients, you would do well to prepare foods from scratch. Even the most innocuous of foods, such as a frozen breaded fish, could have potato as part of the coating.

**Avoid Nightshade Byproducts.** Many packaged foods contain starches of one form or another with potatoes as the source; soups invariably contain tomato products; many herbal or salt-free seasonings have diced green or red peppers and dehydrated tomatoes. Be especially cautious about these disguised nightshade foods in everyday products.

**Yogurt Is Tricky.** Some brands of yogurt contain enough potato starch to cause arthritic pain to flare up. (The starch is used to give "body" to the product.)

**Herbal Beverages.** These are certainly to be preferred to brews containing caffeine, but they may often contain hot peppers! Ordinary herb teas may also have this ingredient.

**Dairy Products.** Certain cheeses contain paprika and this is made from the nightshade pepper! Also, cheeses that have a pink color may also have pepper.

**Baby Foods.** Older folks frequently consume these because of chewing problems. They, too, invariably have potato or tomato products.

**Chocolate.** Best to avoid this confection; not only because of its caffeine (yes, it's there!) and sugar, but because it appears to upset your metabolism when you are on the "no nightshade" diet. It may stimulate more free radicals or interfere with your immune system and negate the benefits of the program.

If you are a nightshade-sensitive person, you may experience a tranquilizing reaction after eating such foods. Do not be lulled into a false sense of security. You will experience an allergic arthritic reaction in a day or so. For many such arthritics, the symptoms become even more severe as the time goes on because of the solanine accumulation in their bodies and the greater destruction of cartilage and tissue. A few moments of comfort are not worth the arthritic pain that follows shortly. Say no to these foods, and you may well say goodbye to your arthritis.

## How Julie R. Overcame Her On-Again, Off-Again Arthritis Pain

As an insurance adjuster, Julie R. had to do a certain amount of traveling. She noticed that when she was on the road for more than a few days, she would develop a recurrence of her painful shoulder and lower back stiffness. But when she remained home, the arthritis disappeared. She was puzzled with this back-and-forth distress. She explained the situation to a company nurse and was told that a clue to the recurring arthritis could be found in her eating habits.

The company nurse said that when Julie R. traveled, she ate in restaurants. Without a doubt, the nightshade foods were causing the reactions. At home, she was careful to avoid such foods and was free of arthritis.

Julie R. was very careful to select dishes without any of the nightshade foods when she made her next trip. Miraculously, she had no arthritis reactions. Apparently, her immune system reacted with the introduction of solanine from the nightshade foods and this triggered off the arthritis. With this knowledge and some careful planning, which called for knowing what went into the foods she ate at restaurants, Julie R. became immune to arthritis.

# HOW TO EXERCISE AWAY ARTHRITIC PAIN

The accumulation of damaging free radicals and molecular fragments can be halted by simple exercise. Basically, the erosion of the cartilage by the harmful fragments can be nipped in the bud when a certain fluid within the joints is present. *Synovial fluid* is a thick and colorless lubricant that surrounds a joint or bursa and fills a tendon sheath. It may well be the antidote to the corrosive free radicals. You need to "wash" out the radicals with the lubrication of synovial fluid. Otherwise, the "dryness" in your cartilage and cells act as a haven for the damaging molecular wastes.

**Exercise Boosts Joint Lubrication.** When you activate your body, your metabolism speeds up the manufacture of the synovial fluid, among other functions. When this anti-arthritic fluid floods into your aching joints, the free radicals are swept up, washed out, thus giving you the flexibility of a youngster. But *only* through simple exercise can the synovial fluid be produced and put to soothing, healing use.

# SIX EXERCISES THAT REJUVENATE YOUR JOINTS AND EASE ARTHRITIS PAIN

*Before You Begin:* If you are taking painkillers, do *not* exercise, you may be hurting yourself without feeling it. Be sure to follow your health practitioner's advice on exercise for your particular condition. *Never* hurt yourself. If any action or motion causes discomfort, then it is best to stop and rest. Never strain yourself or your efforts will cause more harm than good. Ready? Try any or all of these.

1. Water Gymnastics. Swimming is a great conditioner; it utilizes most of your muscles and joints and will release a potent supply of cartilage washing synovial fluid. *Alternative:* If you cannot or will not swim, then take a tip from trainers of athletes—*walk through the water.* Called hydrogymnastics, it helps exercise your limbs, creates a soothing reaction, and will relieve much of your pain if done on a regular basis.
2. Tight Fingers. Tighten your fist. Hold it for the count of ten. Release and stretch your hand wide open as far as possible for another

count of ten. Repeat with your other hand. This helps to loosen up stiff fingers and wrists. Repeat throughout the day.

3. Stiff Spine. Lie face down; insert hands between your chest and floor (or mattress). Gently raise your torso. Try for only an average lift at the start. Hold for the count of ten and slowly lower. Repeat several times. Helps restore better flexibility to a stiff spinal column.

4. Aching Shoulders. Sit or stand. Keep legs comfortably apart. Put one hand on your hip and lean forward slightly from your waist. Slowly swing your free arm toward the floor, then up in front of your other shoulder. Reverse arms and repeat several times. This takes the kinks out of the gnarled, aching shoulders.

5. Rigid Neck, Painful Back. Sit comfortably and cross your right leg over your left leg and gently *(gently, please!)* twist your torso toward your right. Easy does it as you twist your hips to the left as far as comfortably possible without lifting your shoulders. Hold for the count of ten and then return to your starting position. Reverse direction and repeat again. This sitting exercise frees your joints from congestion and boosts circulation so that the synovial fluid is able to dilute and sweep out the ache-causing molecular fragments.

6. Painful Hips, Stiff Lower Spine. Stretch out on your bed, face up. Keep knees bent. Clasp hands behind the nape of your neck. Gently twist your hips to the left as far as is comfortably possible without lifting your shoulders. Hold for the count of ten and return to starting position. Reverse direction and repeat again. This exercise helps unlock the congestion in your lower region, especially around your pelvis. Repeated regularly, it helps restore strength to your skeletal structure and will boost the vigor of your cartilage.

## WHY EXERCISE IS A PAIN-REDUCING ANTIOXIDANT

The various squeezing action of your joints will nourish your cartilage, and the harmful oxidative products will be removed. Oxygen is transported via joint fluid to your cartilage to create an antioxidant condition that reduces and removes arthritic pain.

**Regular Exercise = Freedom from Arthritis.** Exercise becomes an antioxidant when performed regularly. It helps improve the health of your arthritic cartilage. Exercise makes its surface smoother. Bone becomes eburnated or polished with this simple procedure.

## Leaves Wheelchair,
## Becomes a Dancer in Fifteen Days

Painful arthritic spasms so devitalized Barbara U. that in her early forties she had to rely upon the wheelchair in order to get around. Fearing total disability, she sought help from a physical therapist who diagnosed her condition as an excess of oxidative factors which were causing blockages at key joint sites. This was a prime factor in her threatening arthritis.

Barbara U. followed the set of six exercises. Granted, her stiffness had progressed to the degree where she could scarcely bend at the waist to tie her shoe laces, but she was determined to uproot and cast out the cause of the threatening arthritis. She persisted and spent less than fifteen minutes a day with the exercises.

In five days she could walk to the corner store with the greatest of ease. In ten days she could twist and turn in almost all directions. By the end of the fifteenth day her joints had become so youthfully flexible as the arthritis just disappeared, she wanted to prove that she was completely cured and became a dancing teacher. The six exercises had reversed the trend and brought her freedom from the painful arthritis!

**How the Exercise Banished Arthritis.** In just fifteen minutes a day the set of six exercises strengthen the body's supporting ligaments and muscles. They stabilize the joints and bones themselves. They create a biological metabolic reaction that distributes the cleansing synovial fluid so that the burning fragments of free radicals can be extinguished and removed. Inner healing erased the cause of arthritis.

Remember, your exercise should be neither traumatic nor jolting. Let pain be your guide, your warning signal to ease up. Your exercise should be as much as you can comfortably tolerate while doing them, immediately afterwards, and the next morning.

# HEALING YOUR ARTHRITIS WITH WATER

Hydrotherapy is one of the most ancient methods for helping to heal and soothe arthritic pains. Putting it simply, it is water therapy. A relaxing bath or a brisk shower is most soothing to your distress. Hydrotherapy is able to dissolve and disperse the products of inflammation locked in your joints, muscles, and tendons. And you can use hydrotherapy right at home, in your leisure time. There are two forms of water healing and they work almost at once to wash out the irritants that cause arthritis.

1. Heliotherapy. Warm water applications, whether in the form of a soaked towel placed on the aching part, or total immersing of your body in comfortably warm water, are most useful. The warmth will relax muscle spasms, relieve the congestion, and induce a dispersion of the pain-causing fragments.

20-Minute Tub Soak Washes Out Wastes. Just immerse yourself in a tub of comfortably warm water. *Not* hot water, please! All you need do is just let yourself relax. If the bath induces perspiration, it is working. Within 20 minutes, your open pores will help eliminate various kinds of infectious matter, such as urea and other toxic materials. If you prefer, take a brisk, warm shower to wash off clinging wastes and finish with a cooling shower spray to close your pores. *Suggestion:* Enjoy a 20-minute warm tub soak every night and you will not only sleep with less pain, but awaken with more agility since the wastes have been removed from your joints and bones.

2. Cryotherapy. This is also known as cold therapy, and it may date back to the Ice Age, when a primitive human, suffering with a bout of arthritis in the ankles, went across a glacial stream and noticed that the cold water numbed the pain. Today we know that comfortably cool or cold water can help ease the distress of arthritis. It may well be a natural medicine and it is free of money and free of side effects! It's yours for the taking. Cryotherapy via a cooling bath helps increase the viscosity of the blood as well as the peripheral resistance. This helps your heart drive blood throughout your system to wash away irritants.

In particular, cryotherapy sends white corpuscles and increased oxygen into the pockets of your circulatory-skeletal-muscular system. They work to cleanse these sites of infectious bacteria and help reduce inflammation and congestion. Cryotherapy further assists in the elimination of urea, uric acid, and ammonia from the body which can cause your arthritic distress.

## Soak and Shake in Your Cool Tub.

Submerge yourself in a cool tub. Plan to remain for 20 to 30 minutes, but you can do more than just enjoy the cooling relief. You need to shake or move in the cool water-filled tub. In the water, your body loses as much weight as the water it displaces. (*Example:* If you displace five gallons of water, you reduce your weight in water by about 41 pounds.) Notice how your limbs float; your elbows and knees no longer must struggle against the weight of bone and muscle. This means it is much easier for even the most painful of limbs to *gently* exercise while in the cool tub.

*How to Do It:* Just wiggle and shake, twist and turn, jog, dog paddle, swim upstream—use these motions while in the cool tub. When you emerge, you will discover a delightful release from much of your former pain and inflammation. Include cryotherapy exercises as part of your antioxidant arthritis-ending program.

## HOW TO USE ICE TO PUT THE FREEZE ON ARTHRITIC PAIN

You have a powerful pain reliever right in your kitchen freezer—ice. It is the ultimate tool in cryotherapy. It has been found to be extremely beneficial in soothing stubborn arthritic pains.

**How to Use Ice.** Fill an ordinary ice pack with six to ten ice cubes. Put it either slightly above or below the aching joint. Wrap a towel around the ice pack and hold it snugly against the spot for 30 minutes. You will experience coldness, then warming, and finally a numbing. The pain seems to just go away. Repeat several times a day.

**Arthritis in Hands and Feet.** Try a contrast bath. Fill one basin or bowl with ice water, another with comfortably hot water. Place the painful hands or feet first in the hot water for ten minutes then contrast in the ice water for one minute. Continue switching for 30 minutes. You will soon notice how the pain has eased and your hands and feet are much more flexible, thanks to this contrast bath. Remember, finish with cold water for maximum benefits.

When you consider that hydrotherapy (whether warm or cold) has no side effects as does drug therapy, is inexpensive, and boosts the body's own healing processes, you may well appreciate its values.

*Caution:* Folks with diabetes and circulatory ailments such as arteriosclerosis, poor circulation, Raynaud's phenomenon, certain collagen and blood conditions, should use hydrotherapy only under a doctor's supervision.

You need not become vulnerable to the disabling condition of arthritis. Correct your body's metabolism. Follow a "no oxidant" program that uproots and cleanses your joints from irritants and you will be able to have a long and healthy life.

# SUMMARY

1. Distinguish between the two basic forms of arthritis to better understand your personal situation. Take heed of the four warning signs.
2. For many people arthritis is an allergic reaction. Specifically, the four foods of the nightshade family can trigger attacks. Avoid these foods and you may well avoid arthritis.
3. Construction foreman Ben A. conquered his crippling arthritis within six days on a "no nightshade" program.
4. Julie R. was troubled with on-again, off-again arthritis until she followed the "no nightshade" program while dining out. She was soon free of the problem.
5. Six fun-to-do exercises help boost joint lubrication and ease arthritis almost at once.
6. Barbara U. was confined to a wheelchair until she used the antidoxidant exercises and not only was able to walk, but became a dancer!
7. Water, either comfortably warm or cold, can be a natural therapeutic help to ease away arthritic stiffness.
8. Ordinary ice applications can numb and eliminate arthritic pain.

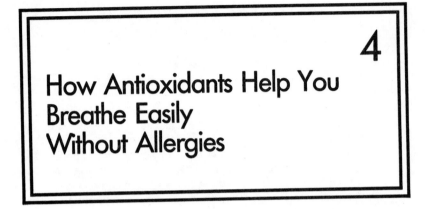

# How Antioxidants Help You Breathe Easily Without Allergies

## 4

For over 31 million people breathing can be an agonizing experience. These people are victims of allergies; that is, free radicals and waste products have entered their bronchial and respiratory systems to clog their breathing apparatus. If you are among those who suffer from allergies, you need to take advantage of antioxidants that will help dissolve and liquefy these molecular fragments, so that your sensitivity is reduced, or even ended. You will then be able to enjoy healthy and youthful breathing.

## WHAT IS AN ALLERGY?

An allergy is a reaction to an accumulation of waste products that include free radicals. These may be taken into your body by inhalation, swallowing or by contact with your skin.

**What Are Common Allergy–Causing Fragments?** Pollens, molds, house dust, animal dander (skin shed by dogs, cats, horses, rabbits), feathers (as in feather pillows), kapok, wool dyes, chemicals used in industry, certain foods and medicines, and insect stings are common allergy-causers. When they enter your body they upset your molecular structure. They damage lipids in the membranes and cause pieces of molecules to break off. These become the accumulative free radicals that bring on allergies through irritation.

**How Do These Wastes Cause Such Reactions?** When the offending substance is absorbed into the bloodstream, it stimulates lymphocytes (small white blood cells) to produce allergic antibodies. These substances react with the offender and produce a reaction which may affect your nose, eyes, lungs, or digestive system. There may be a time delay before such symptoms are noted. Once they happen, they may recur frequently and with more severity each time.

**What Are Typical Allergic Conditions?** Allergic conditions may involve any part or system of the body. Most frequently involved is the bronchial-respiratory system, which brings on conditions such as asthma, hay fever, and rhinitis; there are skin reactions such as atopic eczema, contact dermatitis, and hives (urticaria), to name the most common.

To rebuild immunity you need to bring in antioxidants, whether in the form of nutrients or in breathing methods, as well as some corrections in your diet. You need to bolster your immune forces to resist the corrosive effects of these irritants. Putting it simply, being allergy-free is an inside job!

## FIVE ANTIOXIDANTS THAT WASH OUT ALLERGY–CAUSING IRRITANTS

Wheezing. Itching. Sneezing. Coughing. Weeping. These are symptoms of irritants that are responsible for your particular allergy. They often strike older people and can be so debilitating, that they can make you look and feel older than you really are. Antioxidants are able to call a halt to the irritation of allergies and strengthen your immune system to resist these microscopic invaders. There are five basic antioxidants that work wonders in easing, erasing, and then washing out these molecular fragments. They work speedily in helping you breathe better and healthier. Use any or all of them for your particular needs.

**1. Vitamin A Rebuilds Cellular Integrity.** Dry, rough skin and poor resistance to infection is a symptom of a deficiency in this valuable antioxidant nutrient. Your cells become fragile and vulnerable to the malicious actions of external pollutants. This can trigger allergic reactions.

*How Vitamin A Uses Antioxidant Power.* It protects your tissues, particularly in your respiratory tract, from pollution irritants such as ozone and nitrogen dioxide. Vitamin A rebuilds the integrity of your bronchial cells and tissues, creating a fortress of immunity against the hazards of free radicals.

*How to Use Vitamin A for Allergy Correction.* Select foods such as dark leafy green and deep yellow vegetables; deeply colored fruits such as apricots, cantaloupe, watermelon; other foods such as liver, egg yolk, milk, and butter. An excellent source of Vitamin A is ordinary *cod liver oil,* which contains a concentrated supply of this valuable antioxidant vitamin.

**2. Vitamin C Creates Collagen Power.** Also known as ascorbic acid, it is vital to collagen formation. Collagen is the connective tissue substance that is needed to build immunity to radicals in the form of smoke and pollution. A deficiency in this vitamin causes a breakdown in your cells and a reduction in the amount of red blood cells; also bacterial infections can bring on repeated allergic attacks.

*How Vitamin C Uses Antioxidant Power.* Vitamin C helps to build and regenerate your trillions of cell walls; it helps the manufacture of collagen, the substance that acts as a barrier against harmful toxic fragments. It is able to resist the invasion of offending molecules and granules, especially those that threaten your *mast cells.* Vitamin C has the antioxidant power to get to the root cause of your allergy by strengthening your valuable mast cells. These cells are found in your connective tissue and contain many cytoplasmic granules which are sources of protective secretions to shield you from allergic attacks. Vitamin C, with its antioxidant power, gives strength and vigor to your mast cells so you can develop built-in resistance and inner immunity to allergies.

*How to Use Vitamin C for Allergy Correction.* Vitamin C is found in citrus fruits, mostly in their juices, and in tomato, broccoli, green peppers, raw leafy greens, and white and sweet potatoes in a smaller, but still appreciable degree. Plan to use these sources of vitamin C on a *daily* basis. You need to build resistance *before* you develop an allergic invasion. Enjoy oranges, grapefruits, tangerines, lemons, limes, papaya, strawberries, and cantaloupe, to name a few. Drink their freshly squeezed juices, too, for speedier strengthening of your cells. This is a tasty way to build your immune system with a powerful antioxidant vitamin.

**3. Bioflavonoids Are Natural Antihistamines.** A member of the Vitamin C antioxidant group, *bioflavonoids,* are especially potent in restoring capillary integrity. Bioflavonoids are prime sources of *hesperidin* and *rutin,* a pair of powerful irritant-washers. Found in the stringy or pulpy portions of oranges and particularly grapefruits, these powerful antioxidants are able to maintain blood vessel strength. They are also involved in blood vessel chemistry. Bioflavonoids may well be the most powerful antioxidant available in building immunity to allergies.

*How Bioflavonoids Use Antioxidant Power.* With the use of hesperidin and rutin, the bioflavonoids transport hydrogen throughout the system, boosting the formation of hemoglobin, the distribution of iron, and the development of connective tissues. These reactions cause an antioxidant reaction that helps guard against allergic sensitivities.

*How to Use Bioflavonoids for Allergy Correction.* When you peel a grapefruit or orange be sure to eat the stringy "web" clinging to the rind of the fruit. This part is a powerhouse of valuable bioflavonoids. Just munch it along with the rest of the fruit or add it to a fruit salad. You will boost your inner immunity through the extra fortification of bioflavonoids. A remarkable antioxidant, it is able to protect against proliferation of broken molecules that may form into allergies.

**4. Vitamin E for "Extra" Immunity to Allergy.** Found largely in wheat germ oil, whole grain breads and cereals, peanuts, walnuts, bran and wheat germ, vitamin E is a valuable antioxidant because it keeps your metabolic process in balance. It helps prevent the formation of toxic substances, and works with vitamin A to guard against the destruction of important nutrients. Vitamin E prevents premature reaction of oxygen in the body, protects your breathing system, and cleans out free radicals.

*How Vitamin E Uses Antioxidant Power.* In order for you to be free of allergies you need to have a healthful oxidation or combustion process taking place within each of your cells. Nutrients must not combine in the stomach, intestine, bloodstream, or any other place *before* they reach the cell. If they do combine too soon, combustion takes place to create a waste material that is not only useless, but is also harmful. It could be toxic. It is this form of oxidation that can cause allergic reactions, but this reaction does not happen in the presence of biologically active vitamin E. This nutrient acts as an antioxidant; it prevents oxygen from combining with foods until both are carried in their pure states to the individual cell. Vitamin E uses its antioxidant power to conserve your body's supply of oxygen and keep your tissues more fully oxygenated. This is the natural way to build *internal immunity* through the antioxidant power of vitamin E.

*How to Use Vitamin E for Allergy Correction.* Boost your intake of vegetable oils; wheat germ in any form is most important. Include leafy vegetables, raw nuts, peanuts, soybeans, peas, beans, whole grain breads and cereals. Use them on a regular basis. Do not wait to have an allergic attack before starting to use this antioxidant vitamin. Give your body the necessary working materials that create a balanced oxidation process with the use of the watchdog vitamin E, so that you can not only ease the symptoms of your allergies, but get rid of them, too.

**5. Proper Breathing Technique Can Cause Antioxidant Cleansing.** For the allergic person, breathing can be a chore. In severe cases, you may have the feeling of being suffocated. This is your body's attempt to get rid of the irritants that are to blame for your allergy. You need to give your body a fresh stream of oxygen and it can be done by more effective breathing.

*How Proper Breathing Becomes Antioxidant Power.* Send lifegiving and nutrient-carrying oxygen into your bloodstream with simple daily breathing programs. Since cell rebuilding and cleansing nutrients can reach targets only via the bloodstream on a sea of oxygen, you can readily appreciate the value of deep, rhythmic breathing. You will discover that you will have greater immunity to allergens and the irritation of free radicals if you devote about 30 minutes a day to rhythmic, deep breathing programs. Just breathe in as deeply as you can, hold it for the count of five, then exhale all the way. This will create an antioxidant power that could very well be a healer for your allergies.

*How to Use Breathing for Allergy Correction.* At frequent intervals practice alternate nostril breathing. This appears to maximize the antioxidant reactions of this method. Gently hold one nostril closed by pressing a finger tip against the lower portion. Breathe in through the open nostril; now quickly move finger tip to close the other nostril and breathe out through the just opened nostril. Repeat up to ten minutes a day. This will give you an oxygen reservoir that will balance oxidation so that there will be less risk of fragment accumulation, the cause of many allergies.

Uproot and dislodge the irritating and accumulative elements that are causing your allergic distress. Include one or more of the preceding five antioxidants in your daily lifestyle and you will breathe easier and feel younger, too.

## "Aging" Allergy Victim is Freed
## of Lifelong Distress and Looks Younger

Howard I. was allergic as far back as he could remember. The slightest dust, the merest suggestion of an environmental offender, and he would break out in coughing and sneezing spasms. He could hardly sleep through the night because of recurring bouts with respiratory wheezes and spasms. He looked much older than his actual young age of 52. Medications made him groggy and confused. He might have continued suffering had not a holistic allergist suggested he try the five antioxidant programs as outlined above. They would help erase the cause of the allergy, relieve symptoms, and promote healing.

Because he was desperate, Howard I. planned his daily schedule to include vitamins A, C, E, and the bioflavonoids. He also did the breathing programs. Within five days, much of his coughing and hacking subsided. By the end of nine days, he not only was breathing freely, but his haggard look was gone and he took on a more youthful appearance. The antioxidants had given him a new breath of life! He was healed of his so-called "lifelong" allergy.

# CORRECT CHRONIC COUGHING
# WITH WASTE CLEANSING

Frequent coughing is nature's way of telling you that your breathing apparatus has become clogged with irritating particles. Coughing can be useful in helping to keep your respiratory tract free of excessive fragment buildup, but if they are allowed to cling to your cells, they build up to such an extent that your body reacts with paroxysms of intense coughing. Harsh, painful coughing can cause serious injuries to your rib cage. While an occasional cough is helpful, habitual coughing spells indicate your need to use antioxidant programs to remove these harmful fragments from your cells.

**Six-Step Throat–Soothing Food Program** Be good to your throat and help wash away accumulated debris with this antioxidant program that easily fits into your daily regimen. The goal is to cut down on the supply of wastes quickly. This eases the irritation-producing cough. You will feel youthfully good all over.

1. Use natural seasonings only. Flavorful herbs and spices should replace cell-destroying salt, pepper, mustard, ketchup, and commercial (chemical) seasonings. When you eliminate these assaults on your molecules, you ease the congestion and control deposition of toxic sludge. Almost at once, you will feel a refreshing difference.

2. Avoid temperature extremes in foods, drinks. If the item is too hot, it burns away the cellular coating and renders the molecular interior more vulnerable to attack. If the item is too cold, it congests and tightens your breathing apparatus and this causes the locked molecules to remain frozen and immobile. This will cause cough difficulties and subsequent allergies. *Suggestion:* Let the food or drink be at a comfortable room temperature for better enjoyment and throat pampering.

3. Try fenugreek tea for antioxidant reaction. Available at health food stores and some supermarkets, this aromatic herb of the legume family is a rich source of a mucilaginous substance. This is a powerful antioxidant because it is a mucus solvent and throat cleanser. The slightly sticky viscosity of this tea made from fenugreek seeds will soften and dissolve accumulated and hardened masses of cellular debris. Fenugreek tea is able to soften, dissolve, and wash out the debris. This antioxidant reaction will cleanse your throat and reduce the urge to cough. You'll also build greater resistance to allergies because of the cleansing reaction of this fragrant, licorice-like tea. Drink several cups daily.

4. Increase intake of vitamin C fruits. These fruits are potent cell-scrubbers and also are able to cause formation of collagen, the valuable substance that builds strong cells and tissues. Include oranges, grapefruit, tangerines, papaya, strawberries, cantaloupe (and their juices) in your daily meal program. They impart much needed antioxidant reactions for better breathing.

5. Increase intake of fresh raw juices. Between meals plan to take a freshly prepared raw fruit or vegetable juice. You may make various combinations of different fruits in one drink, or different vegetables for another drink. Do *not* combine fruits and vegetables in the same juice because your enzymatic pattern will clash and the antioxidant process will be thwarted. In highly concentrated form, raw juices are able to soothe your throat and establish a healthier oxidative balance.

6. Salt vapors will soothe and cleanse clogged cells. As an abrasive (ever try it for cleaning stubborn stains?), salt is useful, but healthwise, it helps your throat only when inhaled. If salt is used in foods, it creates an irritating oxidative process that induces allergic re-

actions. You can ease your cough problems by cleansing your clogged cells with a salt vapor treatment. Just add a few tablespoons of salt to a small saucepan of freshly boiled water. Remove the pan and place on a fireproof surface. Stir until salt is dissolved. Put a towel over your head like a tent and slowly inhale the oxygenated salt. Hold your breath for the count of five, then breathe out. Repeat for up to ten minutes. Remove towel tent, spill out water, and relax in a draft-free room. The salt vapors actually scrub away irritating radical fragments. Your freshly washed cells let you breathe better without a hacking cough. *Suggestion:* cleanse your cells with this salt vapor at least once a week. You'll help keep your throat clean and guard against the risk of allergy-causing molecular fragments.

### Conquers Coughing Habit in Four Days

Factory foreman Earl N. J. was so plagued with a coughing habit, he could hardly hold a conversation for more than ten minutes without an irritating outburst. The medical supervisor cautioned that constant abuse to his bronchii could cause permanent distention of his rib cage. To help him counter this undesirable habit, the supervisor suggested a simple six-step antioxidant program. Within two days, Earl N. J. cut his coughing spells in half. In four days, he jokingly remarked he didn't know what a cough was! This antioxidant program had given him a clean bill of health . . . free of allergies!

## TWO EVERYDAY FOODS THAT HAVE ANTIOXIDANT POWER TO BUILD IMMUNITY TO ALLERGIES

Toxic wastes or free radicals can cause sensitivization of your breathing apparatus. Even slight amounts of ordinary dust or floral pollen (such as in hay fever) can bring on a serious attack. These molecular fragments in the form of molds are usually microscopic in size. Fungus-like, they fasten themselves to your bronchial tubes and soon multiply to the point that you become victim to *respiratory pollution.* Slight amounts of ordinary dust can cause a choking and weeping reaction. To help build immunity, you will discover that two special but everyday foods have antioxidant powers that make them comparable to medicine. And they're all-natural, too!

1. Antioxidant Power of Garlic. This miracle vegetable is a prime source of two ingredients, *allicin* and *alliin,* which cause antioxidant reactions that can build your immunity to allergens. You need to use garlic on a daily basis to develop this immunity. Try this simple method:

*Garlic Juice.* Press the juice from two or three garlic cloves into a glass of freshly prepared vegetable juice. Stir. Drink slowly. *Careful!* Just a few drops of the garlic juice will be enough for the antioxidant reaction.

Drink up to two glasses of garlic juice daily and you will create a storehouse of antioxidant resistance to the invasion of harmful substances that are to blame for allergies. It is like having an immune station within your system!

2. Antioxidant Power of Horseradish. This Old World flavoring for food has been used for centuries to clear stuffed noses and promote youthful breathing. Often, it works within minutes. Horseradish contains antiseptic properties that are able to cauterize the accumulated molecular fragments and slough them out of your respiratory tract. By trying this method, you can breathe easier and freer. And you can build inner immunity to avoid allergies in the future.

*How to Use:* Just add one-quarter of a teaspoon of horseradish to a glass of vegetable juice to create the antioxidant effect. Or, add the same amount to a plate of raw or cooked vegetables. *Careful:* Horseradish is volatile, more so than garlic, hence its dynamic effectiveness in clearing away wastes so speedily. Use just a small amount. Within minutes after you partake of horseradish you will experience a respiratory refreshment that will make you feel youthfully healthy again. It is proof of the antioxidant working powers of this food.

Plan to use both garlic and horseradish as part of your daily meal plan to accelerate your powers of immunity against allergies.

## Wins Lifelong Allergy Battle by Using Two Foods

Use of drugs, moving about for climate changes, even hypnotherapy failed to release schoolteacher Natalie McD. from her lifelong enslavement to the throat-racking agony of allergic attacks. Even the slightest amount of dust made her have a runny nose and begin sneezing, coughing, and choking until she thought she would suffocate! She might have continued her downward trend to eventual confinement had not a nutritionally aware allergist recommended the antioxidant properties of both garlic and horseradish. He recommended she try the programs on a daily basis. Desperate, Natalie McD. followed the plan. She drank four glasses of garlic-vegetable juice daily and took about one-quarter to one-half teaspoon of horseradish daily. Within one day, the antioxidant foods helped her breathe better. Within four days, her formerly "hopeless" and "lifelong" allergy had been conquered. She won the battle, thanks to the antioxidant action of cleansing her bronchial-respiratory tract of allergy-provoking irritants.

## HOW TO LENGTHEN YOUR "SHORTNESS OF BREATH"

Breathlessness indicates that your larynx (voice box at the entrance to your windpipe) and related respiratory organs have become clogged with destructive free radicals. You may find it difficult to climb a reasonable amount of stairs; you may experience tightness of breath when carrying bundles, when excited, when getting up, and when performing many chores. You need to clean your larynx and "lengthen" your "shortness" of breath. A simple antioxidant program that washes your lungs, when performed three times daily, can give you the improved breathing you so desperately crave.

### Three Simple Breath–Improving Antioxidant Exercises

1. Starting Position: Stand with your feet comfortably spaced, knees slightly bent. Clasp hands, palms together, close to your chest. *Action:* Press your hands together, breathe in very deeply, and hold for the count of five. Loosen hands and breathe out. Repeat at least five times.

2. Starting Position: Stand with your feet slightly apart, knees slightly bent. Grip fingers and arms close to your chest. *Action:* Pull hard and breathe in completely, exhale completely, as you try to pull your fingers apart. Repeat at least five times.

3. Starting Position: Sit comfortably on a chair. Space your feet about four inches apart. Bend forward. Place your hands on the insides of your opposite knees. *Action:* Breathe in deeply while you try to press knees together while holding them apart with your hands. Breathe out deeply as you try again. Repeat at least five times.

*Benefits:* This oxygenation helps restore the integrity of the DNA-RNA genetic code nucleus in your cells. Since DNA-RNA components have built-in repair mechanisms that depend upon nutrition via oxygenation, these easy programs will strengthen them so they can give you immunity to allergic refuse.

*Suggestion:* Plan to follow these antioxidant actions daily (total time is only less than ten minutes) to give you the resistance you need.

### Enjoys "Complete" Breathing with Antioxidant Exercises

Selma A. N. felt sharp "constriction" when she climbed atop a small foot stool to reach for an item on a top shelf. Breathing was difficult. Climbing a few steps provoked a painful coughing spasm, a discolored face, and agonizing sputters for precious air. She asked a local physical therapist for help. He recommended the preceding three-step antioxidant exercise. Selma A. N. followed them easily. Within two days, she had regained complete breathing ability. She could now climb several flights without shortness of breath.

Free yourself of the threat of choking by using antioxidant foods and therapeutic programs to help correct the oxidative processes in your system. You will be able to breathe with youthful comfort when equilibrium has been established. And you can do this all at home within a short time.

## IMPORTANT POINTS

1. Troubled with wheezing, itching, sneezing, coughing, weeping? Ease and cast out allergy-causing irritants with the use of any or all five antioxidants. You'll breathe easier almost at once.
2. Howard I. conquered a lifelong allergy by using the five antioxidants, saving his job and his health, too.
3. A six-step throat-soothing food program helps overcome stubborn coughs.
4. Earl N. J. conquered his coughing habit on the six-step antioxidant program within four days.
5. Garlic and horseradish are traditional antioxidant foods that help build immunity to allergies.

6. Natalie McD. won lifelong freedom and future immunity from allergies by using just two foods.
7. Permanent immunity against allergy is possible with the three simple breath-improving antioxidant exercises.
8. Selma A. N. "lengthened" her shortness of breath with easy exercises.

# How Antioxidants Build Immunity to Arteriosclerosis

Also known as hardening of the arteries, the condition of *arteriosclerosis* is triggered by an accumulation of fat and cholesterol on the blood vessel walls of your cardiovascular system. It is a "whole body" condition that has its beginnings in the weakening of your immune system. Namely, your body has been made vulnerable to the accumulation of excess amounts of these fatty deposits. If allowed to remain, this overload of fat deposits may injure your blood vessel walls and clog up your arteries to the extent that you could be vulnerable to a stroke or heart attack. Permanent effects could be paralysis, brain damage, even death.

The danger signals of arteriosclerosis are high blood pressure, overweight, diabetes, and a family history of heart trouble. These are just some of the warning signs that should be heeded in order to guard against the threat of arteriosclerosis.

## CHOLESTEROL—TRIGLYCERIDE FREE RADICALS ARE TO BLAME

Two principal types of fat in the bloodstream, cholesterol and triglyceride, are closely associated with arteriosclerosis and heart attacks. They may be considered "aging" forms of free radicals.

**Irritant Reaction of Fatty Radicals.** When in excessively high amounts, these fatty radicals become irritants to artery walls, particularly to damaged ones (damaged by the fragments of molecules and misshapen cross-linked cells), and contribute to the formation of plaques. These are the dangerously large and connected cross-links that can cause serious repercussions. These fatty, free radicals are the root cause of arteriosclerosis, the so-called "old person's condition." Surely, if your goal is to live a long and healthy life, you want it to be free of this arterial hardening that can be a block to your objective of longevity.

With the use of antioxidants you can help control the levels of cholesterol-triglyceride in your bloodstream and have a youthful cardiovascular system.

You could plan to go on a low animal fat program, and be partially benefitted since cholesterol-triglyceride radicals are formed almost solely out of animal foods. You could even eliminate *all* animal foods. This would not be especially wise since you do need a minimal amount of fat to act as a means of transporting vitamins and minerals and to participate in various metabolic processes. A reduction of animal fats would be helpful, but you are still at risk of having an overload of fatty, free radicals in your system. The idea is for your body to achieve a metabolic balance by which antioxidant foods are able to metabolize and keep fat levels at a safe ratio.

In brief, not everyone who eats a lot of fat and cholesterol gets arteriosclerosis. Nor does everyone who has a heart attack have an excessively high cholesterol count.

**How Cholesterol is Kept in Control.** Your body closely monitors the production of this fat so that when you eat more cholesterol, your metabolism produces less cholesterol to keep the amount available in the body constant. Conversely, if you eat less cholesterol, then your body makes more. The key to maintaining inner control is in the availability of antioxidants that act as "watchdogs" in guarding against overload.

## ANTIOXIDANTS BOOST PRODUCTION OF VALUABLE HDLS

Cholesterol does not exist in your bloodstream as a single entity. It is dispatched as a component of carriers called *lipoproteins*. One is called the *low-density lipoprotein* (LDL), which is regarded as the harmful fatty radical. The second is called the *high-density lipoprotein* (HDL), which is regarded as the helpful and lifesaving type of fat. It has been noted that the higher the level of HDLs, the better your immunity against cardiovascular distress.

### How Antioxidants Create Immune-Building HDLs.

You need to give your metabolism an abundance of antioxidant foods so that you can have a higher level of these vulnerable immune-building HDLs. Your goal is to guard against *oxidation* of the cell membrane. It is this oxidative process that causes an increase in the harmful LDLs. But with the presence of antioxidants, this deterioration is controlled and there is a corresponding increase of the immune-building HDLs.

*Problem:* During the intake of average fatty foods, your metabolism works to help burn up the fat to guard against overload. Yet, oxidation still occurs because of the presence of free radicals. These tiny molecular particles or compounds containing unpaired, highly charged electrons are very unstable. They combine with the fats from foods to form peroxides which are caustic to cell membranes. This sets off a chain reaction that creates many more free radicals. Soon, your body's defenses become weakened. More of the harmful low-density lipoproteins accumulate. These are threats to your very being. Your immune system becomes weak and the stage is set for arteriosclerosis and related cardiovascular illnesses.

*Solution:* Antioxidants have the power to foil the free radicals' destruction of cell membranes; they help to cause an oxidation of the rancid fats and free radicals and help restore the necessary higher levels of the valuable high-density lipoproteins. With antioxidants, there is greater built-in protection or autoimmunity against the threat of cholesterol-triglyceride overload.

## THREE ANTIOXIDANTS THAT GIVE YOU IMMUNITY TO ARTERIOSCLEROSIS

While it is certainly wise to follow a reasonably fat-controlled diet, it is also helpful to give your body a supply of the immune-building antioxidants found in three specific food groups. They have the unique ability of helping to create a fortress of resistance against cholesterol-triglyceride asphyxiation and strengthens the inner cellular structure that requires more high-density lipoproteins. You will find these three antioxidants in everyday foods; they are available as supplements, too, which should be used under the supervision of your health practitioner.

1. **Vitamin C as a Fat-Washing Antioxidant.** Its powerful antioxidizing reaction takes place *inside* the cell, right in the fatty fluid.

As vitamin C acts to dissolve the fatty, free radicals, it creates two compounds, *dehydroascorbic acid* and *2,3-diketogulonic acid,* which are believed to be valuable in maintaining strong and disease-free cells. These two compounds are powerful immune-building substances that can protect you against life-threatening conditions.

In particular, vitamin C beefs up your immune system by increasing the activity of lymphocytes; these are white blood cells responsible for producing antibodies to make you immune to infection. Vitamin C increases the number of receptor sites on a lymphocyte's membrane so it can easily latch on to a fatty, free radical and prepare for its removal. You need vitamin C to make an abundance of valuable immune-building and fat-dissolving lymphocytes. It is this antioxidant reaction that may well offer more resistance to the fatty overload of arteriosclerosis than could a controlled diet!

*Sources of Antioxidant Vitamin C.* Vitamin C is present in all citrus fruits and their fresh juices; also in many green vegetables such as green peppers. Plan to use these sources on a daily basis. Remember, vitamin C is *not* stored in the system, so to give yourself maximum antioxidant and immunity protection against arteriosclerosis, include these foods in your menu just about every single day.

**2. Vitamin E Helps Boost HDL Levels.** The key to cholesterol-triglyceride control is, of course, a fat-controlled diet. But this can work only if you are able to maintain a higher level of high-density lipoproteins or HDLs. This is made possible with the use of vitamin E—a valuable antioxidant. It is a fat-soluble nutrient that helps dissolve excess fats, but tends to cause an increase in the valuable HDLs. Picture the cell membrane as a sandwich of fatty layers with vitamin E in the center, guarding against fatty oxidation. This vitamin tends to soak up the free radicals; this prevents oxidation of the cell membrane and allows for an increase in important HDLs.

Vitamin E also extends the life of the red blood cells, which might otherwise become aged because of the cholesterol-triglyceride fatty radical accumulation.

It is this reaction that builds your immunity to the risks of arteriosclerosis. Vitamin E has a stabilizing effect on the cell membranes. Picture it this way: the cell membrane consists of lipids (fats) and proteins. The lipids function like an oily sea containing proteins. Compare it to cooking oil: as you heat or cool it, the consistency is changed. The lipid sea reacts the same to temperature change. To create an antioxidant reaction, you need to monitor these changes by measuring the movement of the protein molecules. The thicker the sea, the slower the movement of the molecules. The thinner the sea, the faster they will move.

Vitamin E influences the fluidity of the membrane much in the same way as does the temperature. Vitamin E prods the proteins to move more freely. It is this increased fluidity that reduces the stickiness of blood platelets and this is a powerful help in building immunity to arteriosclerosis and in correcting the fatty overload, too. Vitamin E uses this antioxidant method to keep your blood fat levels in check.

*Sources of Antioxidant Vitamin E.* Most vegetable oils, particularly wheat germ oil, all seeds; leafy vegetables; raw nuts; peanuts; legumes such as soybeans, peas, beans; whole grain breads and cereals.

### 3. Selenium as a Valuable Antioxidant. Live longer and healthier with selenium? It is possible when we recognize that this powerful mineral acts as an antioxidant to prevent the potential mutagenic effects of certain compounds. It helps to produce a special enzyme, *glutathione peroxidase,* that turns harmful peroxide radicals into neutral water and then washes this water out of the system. Selenium works *within* the cells. It is able to attack the cross-links of glued-together large molecules, dissolve their fatty radicals, and prepare them for elimination.

Selenium helps keep cell breakage in check long enough so that a damaged and fat-filled cell is able to be repaired and have its chromosomes strengthened to give immunity to arteriosclerosis and other threatening conditions.

Basically, when your cells suffer chromosomal damage, they may become malignant; the free radicals that split off and cause fatty overload may also become involved with some malignancy unless the damage is repaired before the cell divides. Selenium is an antioxidant nutrient that delays cell division (mitosis) and becomes involved in DNA repair. It then helps dispose of toxic wastes and fatty fragments that could otherwise form complexes and blood clots. Selenium is one of the lesser-known, but increasingly important, trace minerals that can give you immunity as well as recovery from the risks of arteriosclerosis.

*Sources of Antioxidant Selenium.* This trace mineral is found in the bran and germs of whole grain cereals, broccoli, onions, garlic, tomatoes, and tuna.

## Reverses Arteriosclerosis Threat in Six Days

When Michael F. was told he had a dangerously high level of blood fat and that arteriosclerosis was increasing at a rapid rate, he had to act quickly. While a fat-controlled diet was helpful, he still kept churning more cholesterol-triglyceride levels than his body could accommodate. He sought the help of an internist who used a total body approach, meaning treatment of the problem by treating the whole person. In Michael's case, he needed to build immunity and protection with the use of antioxidants.

He was told to boost intake of the three more powerful fat-dissolving antioxidants, vitamins C, E, and selenium. A simple menu plan featuring these nutrients did the trick. Within four days a reading showed his blood fats had gone almost one-half down the dangerous level. By the end of the sixth day the antioxidants had brought the fats under such control, via increased high-density lipoprotein fortification, he was free of arteriosclerosis. Michael's internist said he had actually "washed away the fats." The antioxidants deserved the credit, maintained Michael, who was free of the danger of life-threatening arteriosclerosis.

# THE ANTIOXIDANT OIL THAT WASHES YOUR ARTERIES

At health food stores, most supermarkets, and many local groceries you can pick up a supply of sunflower seed oil. It is a highly concentrated source of *polyunsaturates,* essential fatty acids and antioxidants. In combination, these elements act like "dynamite" in dislodging stubborn clumps of cholesterol that might otherwise squeeze and choke your arteries and threaten your life.

**Magic Antioxidant Ingredient.** Sunflower seed oil is a prime source of *linoleic acid,* the one essential fatty acid that works like an antioxidant in guarding against buildup of rancid fats in and upon your arteries. This antioxidant ingredient keeps cholesterol wastes soft and manageable, washing them out when required. Linoleic acid uses its antioxidant powers to guard against overload of hard waste deposits that could give rise to age-causing arteriosclerosis.

*How to Use:* In any recipe calling for oil, just substitute sunflower seed oil. Also, mix two parts of this antioxidant oil with one part of apple cider vinegar and use as a salad dressing. Whenever possible replace butter with oil. You may also blenderize two tablespoons of oil with one glass of fresh vegetable juice. Drink it slowly. (The enzymes in the juice will accelerate the antioxidant cleansing action.) For around-the-clock internal antioxidant action, plan to take from four to six tablespoons of sunflower seed oil throughout the day.

## BREWER'S YEAST: POWERFUL ANTIOXIDANT FOR CLEANSING ARTERIES

What is brewer's yeast? It is the dried, pulverized cells of the yeast plant, a powerful concentrate of valuable nutrients that work in harmony to create an antioxidant reaction. It is one of the rare meatless foods that contains nearly all essential amino acids, making it a valuable protein source. A bonus is that brewer's yeast has no fats (which are sources of cholesterol-triglyceride accumulation); its greatest bonus may be in its high concentration of an unusual and little known trace mineral—*chromium*. This can become a powerful antioxidant to keep your arteries young and flexible.

**How Brewer's Yeast Performs Antioxidant Reaction.** Chromium stimulates the *glucose tolerance factor* (GTF) in your system, helping to break up and dissolve the excessive cholesterol-triglyceride overload. This eases the risk of artery clogging. In effect, this antioxidant power is able to wash out excessive fat-sludge, keeping your trillions of cells and tissues in youthful health.

**How to Use Brewer's Yeast.** Available at most health food stores, some pharmacies, and supermarkets, plan to use brewer's yeast daily. Mix one tablespoon into a glass of vegetable juice. Blenderize. Sip slowly. Or else, add a tablespoon of yeast to a kettle of brown rice while still cooking. Include it in soups, stews, baked loaves, casseroles. Add to homemade pancakes, omelets, breads, casseroles. Plan to have from four to six tablespoons daily. You will be supercharging your metabolic system with valuable antioxidants that help keep your fat levels in a proper balance and your arteries in youthful condition.

### Lowers Cholesterol, Cleanses Bloodstream in Nine Days

Troubled by an excessive cholesterol reading, office supervisor Edna Z. went on a low fat diet. Her hematologist (blood specialist) noted the cholesterol levels were still undesirably high. Edna Z. was told to take up to six tablespoons of brewer's yeast daily, in juices and in various recipes. Edna Z. followed this program. Within six days the antioxidant reaction had caused a welcome drop in blood fat readings. By the end of the ninth day on this antioxidant program, she was given happy news. She had a healthy cholesterol–triglyceride level. The valuable high-density lipoproteins were increased and acted as defenses against arteriosclerosis. She was as healthy as a youngster!

## GARLIC AS A SUPER ANTIOXIDANT FOOD

The fragrant, sometimes pungent, but always effective vegetable, garlic, is one of the most powerful antioxidants available. It can prevent plaque formation in arteries and create immunity against the threat of arteriosclerosis and related heart disorders.

The reason here is that garlic contains allicin. This is an active sulfur-containing antioxidant that changes into *diallyldisulphide* in your system. This ingredient is able to reduce lipid levels in your bloodstream and work swiftly to raise valuable HDLs, which are protectors against arteriosclerosis.

Allicin has a marked effect on certain antioxidant processes of synthesis, or breakdown of lipids in the liver. And you know that excessive lipids (fatty substances such as triglycerides and cholesterol) in the arteries are a major risk of arteriosclerosis and cardiovascular disorders.

With the use of garlic on a daily basis as a seasoning (just two or three cloves a day appear to create the needed antioxidant reaction), you should build strong immunity to many age-causing ailments.

## FITNESS IS A POWERFUL ANTIOXIDANT

Simple exercises ranging from daily walking to more vigorous calisthenics can set off an antioxidant reaction. Your goal is to use aerobic exercise, one that floods your system with oxygen, to help put life into the antioxidant process.

Try (doctor-approved) jogging, hiking, tennis, handball, squash, golf, bicycling, rowing, swimming, roller skating, or table tennis. Try dancing. (Yes, it's a great antioxidant exercise, and fun, too.) Try walking upstairs, bowling, mowing your lawn, badminton, gardening. These are enjoyable and recreational activities. Include them in your antioxidant feeding program for overall health.

### Simple Program Sparks Antioxidant Reaction to Rejuvenate Arteries

Lab technician Phil O'Q. felt his vitality slipping through his fingers. He complained of increasing fatigue. Breathing was difficult. His skin color was sallow. At times, his hands trembled. His heartbeat was irregular. Thinking became fuzzy. His memory was so poor, he forgot appointments which created furor among his superiors.

Fortunately, the company cardiovascular physician recognized the symptoms as arterial clogging because of a defect in antioxidant action. The doctor prescribed a low fat program, and consumption of antioxidant foods such as selenium and garlic, but he explained that the most effective antioxidant would be exercise.

Phil O'Q. was told to walk at least 60 minutes daily, and work out at least another 60 minutes daily with any aerobic oxygenating activity from the preceding list. Following the program, Phil expressed doubts that this could help improve his condition. But before long, his doubts turned to amazement.

Within eight days, he perked up. His energy doubled. His breathing was healthy. His hands were steady; his heartbeat strong. His thinking was as good as that of a youngster. Another blood exam showed clean arteries, hence his youthful restoration. Thanks to the antioxidant action of oxygenating exercise, he was totally healthy again!

# CORRECT FATTY OVERLOAD WITH WEIGHT CONTROL

Antioxidants are able to revive your cells and wash out fat, if you cooperate with weight control. Otherwise, excessive fats create *hyperlipidemia.* That is, surplus fatty deposits spill through the blood system and stick to your arteries, inside and outside.

*Problem:* Formation of grayish-white plaques with lipid-filled centers by fibrous caps and stiffened by sediment deposits can occur. These wastes protrude from the arterial wall and tend to group together.

If antioxidant energy is sapped by overload of weight, there could follow a clumping of platelets (blood components that cause clotting) around a break in the surface of the arterial inner wall. These platelet wastes are glued together with fibrous tissue to form dangerous plaque. If plaque attaches to the walls of your arteries, you run the risk of cardiovascular problems. So you can recognize the importance of shedding excess weight; not just for basic health, but for having younger arteries.

**"Clean" Vs. "Unclean" Fats for Youthful Arteries.** You *can* continue to enjoy most of your favorite foods, but with some adjustments. Plan to have more "clean" and less "unclean" fats. Following are some general guidelines.

**"Clean" Fats That Promote Antioxidant Action.** These include: poultry foods, but without the skin; egg whites; breads made with a minimum of saturated fats; biscuits, muffins, and griddle cakes that use liquid oil as a shortening; pasta products with liquid oil as a dressing; tomato sauce made *without* animal fats (read labels). Enjoy cakes, pies, pastries, made *without* animal fats, *without* sugar, and *only* with whole grain flour. Enjoy margarines; liquid oil shortenings; salad dressings; and mayonnaise but only if they contain polyunsaturated vegetable oils that act as antioxidants. Again, read the labels.

These foods give you the fat taste you want, but because they are polyunsaturated they boost the antioxidant action and do not cling to your arteries. So you can have your cake and eat it, too. (Provided it has no animal fats!)

**"Unclean" Fats Block Antioxidant Action.** Heavily marbled and fatty meats, organ meats, breads made with animal fats, commercial mixes containing animal fats, whole milk (switch to skim) products, coconut oil (high in saturated fat), lard, meat fat, hydrogenated margarines, and any fried foods all have fatty wastes that block antioxidant action so that fats are deposited in and on your arteries. This may cause eventual choking of your vital arteries.

Make these simple dietary adjustments with almost no sacrifice in taste (lean meats have great flavor and are healthier for you) and you will have a vigorous antioxidant action that will keep your arteries clean and healthy. Your weight will drop daily until you reach your desired levels. Keep you weight under control and your antioxidant process active and you will have a long and healthy life.

## Loses Weight, Cleans Arteries, Given Longer Life

Fighting the battle of the bulge made Jean LaK. so upset she succumbed to compulsive eating binges. Not only was she an unsightly 235 pounds, with expanding hips and thighs, but her bariatrician (doctor-specialist in obesity) checked her over and found she was on the brink of a serious case of arteriosclerosis.

He put her on the simple "clean" vs. "unclean" antioxidant food program. Desperate to lose weight, Jean LaK. followed the diet. Within eighteen days, she shed some 16 pounds and lost four inches from her girth. By the end of nine weeks, she had slimmed down to 140 pounds and had a 30-inch waist. Shortly afterwards, she was a youthfully slim 118 pounds and had a 24-inch waist. The antioxidant action had cleansed her arteries, and now Jean LaK. was given hope for a longer and healthier life. Antioxidants were allowed to rebuild her health when she lost weight and controlled fatty intake.

Build natural immunity against arteriosclerosis and related cardiovascular disorders with the use of antioxidants. These all-natural miracle workers have the ability to guard against fatty buildup and establish your internal equilibrium so that you can have young arteries and a young lifestyle, too!

# IN REVIEW

1. Be aware of the problem of hardening of the arteries, which is traced to cholesterol-triglyceride buildup. Risky free radicals cause this cardiovascular distress.
2. Antioxidants help produce valuable high-density lipoproteins (HDLs) which keep fatty, radical wastes under control. They become the key to regulation of fats in your system.
3. Three antioxidants, vitamin C, vitamin E, and selenium help give you immunity to arteriosclerosis.

4. Michael F. reversed his arteriosclerosis threat in three days with the use of three fat-dissolving antioxidants.
5. Sunflower seed oil is a powerful antioxidant that controls cholesterol levels.
6. Brewer's yeast contains several natural ingredients that exert a powerful antioxidant reaction to keep cholesterol-triglyceride levels in check.
7. Edna Z. lowered her cholesterol levels and cleansed her bloodstream of dangerous free radicals within nine days with brewer's yeast.
8. Garlic contains allicin, which is one of the most amazing antioxidants available from a natural source. Include garlic in your diet.
9. Include fitness as a means of oxygenating your system. Phil O'Q. sparked this antioxidant reaction with easy exercises and rejuvenated his arteries.
10. Plan menu around "clean" vs. "unclean" fats to enable antioxidants to keep your arteries clean.
11. Correct your weight to boost the antioxidant process. Jean LaK. lost excess weight and was soon free of arteriosclerosis.

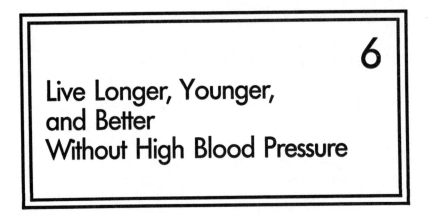

# Live Longer, Younger, and Better Without High Blood Pressure

**6**

You can build immunity to the condition of high blood pressure (also called *hypertension*) with the use of antioxidants found in specific foods. With this built-in protective factor, you will be able to enjoy a long and healthy life free from the threat of a dangerous cardiovascular attack related to elevated blood pressure.

To better understand how to use antioxidants for this protection, it is helpful to become familiar with the definition of blood pressure.

## WHAT IS HIGH BLOOD PRESSURE?

Blood pressure is the force of blood against the walls of the arteries and veins caused by the heart as it pumps blood to every part of the body.

When arterioles (the small arteries that regulate blood pressure) contract, blood cannot easily pass through them. When this happens the heart must pump harder to push the blood through. This increased pushing raises the blood pressure in the arteries. If the blood pressure rises above normal and remains elevated, the result is high blood pressure or hypertension.

**What Is the Problem?** High blood pressure adds to the workload of the heart and arteries. This may contribute to heart failure and arteriosclerosis. The narrowed blood vessels may not be able to deliver enough oxygen to the body's organs and tissues.

**Enlarges Heart.** When the heart is forced to work harder than normal for a long period of time, it tends to enlarge. A slightly enlarged heart may function well, but a heart that is very much enlarged has a difficult time keeping up with the demands on it.

**Wear and Tear.** Arteries and arterioles, too, show the wear and tear of high blood pressure. Eventually, they become hardened, less elastic, and scarred. High blood pressure accelerates this process.

**Life-Threatening Risks.** Hardened or narrowed arteries may not be able to deliver the amount of blood that the body's organs need to function properly. There is also the risk that a blood clot may lodge in a narrowed artery, depriving part of the body of its normal blood supply. Three of the vital organs often damaged are the heart, brain, and kidneys.

**How Widespread Is This Condition?** High blood pressure affects about 35 million Americans, or one out of every six adults. It causes 20,000 deaths annually. It is called a "silent killer" because it normally has no symptoms. To know if you have high blood pressure, you need to have it checked by your doctor. A simple examination uses a sphygmomanometer. This is a rubber cuff that is placed around your arm and then inflated with air. Your doctor listens with a stethoscope to the sound of the blood pushing through the artery. While listening and watching a gauge, your doctor records two measurements: the pressure of blood flow when the heart beats (systolic pressure) and the pressure of the flow of blood between heartbeats (diastolic pressure).

**What is "Safe" Blood Pressure?** Your doctor records both numbers as blood pressure measurements; 120/80 is generally considered safe. The first number listed is the *systolic* pressure (heart beating; the second number is the *diastolic* pressure (between beats). *Caution:* The more difficult it is for the blood to flow, the higher the numbers. If they are much higher than the 120/80 safety guideline, you need to plan a program of adjustments in your lifestyle to help bring down these figures.

## MOLECULAR DISCARDS CAUSE INCREASE IN PRESSURE

An accumulation of free radicals can result in a destruction of the healthy cells that make up your arteries and arterioles. Ordinary blood pressure can be withstood by these pipelines of your cardiovascular system, but when the corrosive molecular discards cause an erosion of your vein and artery walls, this weakening causes a distortion of the force of blood against these walls. These molecular discards or free radicals become blockages. The blood must pump harder and this could cause serious cardiovascular distress.

**Why the Radical Buildup?** The major villain here is salt or sodium chloride. This seasoning causes an inflammatory reaction upon your millions of cells, leading to breakage and destruction. Many of them become fragments that float in the bloodstream and cause mischief in the form of high blood pressure. At the same time, the accumulation of these free radicals create a hydraulic reaction by blocking the transport of vital fluids in your circulatory system. Even if salt is consumed in smaller amounts and for a brief period of time, it can still cause this elevation in pressure that may have serious repercussions. Antioxidants are destroyed in the presence of salt. To help build immunity to high blood pressure, you need to curtail and eliminate the use of salt in all forms.

**Your Lifesaving Goal.** Salt elimination is your first goal, but at the same time, you need to boost your intake of potassium. This mineral has an antioxidant reaction that washes out the molecular fragments and builds immunity to high blood pressure. To begin, you need to follow this program that is outlined next (see the chart on p. 65-71).

## HOW TO AVOID SALT TO PROMOTE STRONGER ANTIOXIDANT POWER

Because you have probably been using salt over a long (too long) period of time, your taste buds want a tang of excitement. You can still have spicy satisfaction by using flavorful herbs and spices in place of salt. Other ways to enjoy natural flavors without salt include:

- Use lemon and lime wedges on many foods. These tart fruits are just about sodium-free. You'll enjoy a fragrant, tangy flavor that makes up for the absence of salt.
- Avoid salt in cooking and at your table.
- Use salt-free butter or margarine.

- Most canned, frozen, dehydrated, processed foods and beverages are high in sodium. Read labels. Select salt-free products.
- Many breakfast foods are high in sodium; others are low. Again, read labels and make a wise choice.
- Homemade salad dressings (oil-vinegar-herbs) contain little sodium. Commercial dressings and mayonnaise are high in sodium.
- Most fresh meats and poultry products are low in sodium, but processed meats (ham, bacon, sausage, frankfurters, and so forth) are high in this pressure-raising substance.
- Similarly, fresh fish is rather low in sodium, but processed fish often has added salt. The label tells all.

## SODIUM–POTASSIUM–CALORIE COUNTER

This diet chart has been prepared for people who must watch the sodium, potassium and or calories in the food they eat. The figures are listed for average portions of food commonly eaten . . . to make it easier for you to follow your doctor's instructions.

| Meat and Poultry* | Portion | Sodium (mg.) | Potassium (mg.) | Calories |
|---|---|---|---|---|
| Bacon | 1 strip (1 oz.) | 71 | 16 | 156 |
| Beef | | | | |
|   Corned Beef (canned) | 3 slices | 803 | 51 | 184 |
|   Hamburger | ¼ lb. | 41 | 382 | 224 |
|   Pot Roast (rump) | ½ lb. | 43 | 309 | 188 |
|   Sirloin Steak | ½ lb. | 57 | 545 | 260 |
| Chicken (broiler) | 3½ oz. | 78 | 320 | 151 |
| Duck | 3½ oz. | 82 | 285 | 326 |
| Frankfurter (all beef) | ⅛ lb. | 550 | 110 | 129 |
| Ham | | | | |
|   Fresh | ¼ lb. | 37 | 260 | 126 |
|   Cured, butt | ¼ lb. | 518 | 239 | 123 |
|   Cured, shank | ¼ lb. | 336 | 155 | 91 |

| Meat and Poultry* | Portion | Sodium (mg.) | Potassium (mg.) | Calories |
|---|---|---|---|---|
| Lamb | | | | |
|   Shoulder Chop (1) | ½ lb. | 72 | 422 | 260 |
|   Rib Chop (2) | ½ lb. | 68 | 398 | 238 |
|   Leg Roast | ¼ lb. | 41 | 246 | 96 |
| Liver | | | | |
|   Beef | 3½ oz. | 86 | 325 | 136 |
|   Calf | 3½ oz. | 131 | 436 | 141 |
| Pork | | | | |
|   Loin Chop | 6 oz. | 52 | 500 | 314 |
|   Spareribs (3 or 4) | 3½ oz. | 51 | 360 | 209 |
|   Sausage (link or bulk) | 3½ oz. | 740 | 140 | 450 |
| Turkey | 3½ oz. | 40 | 320 | 268 |
| Veal | | | | |
|   Cutlet | 6 oz. | 46 | 448 | 235 |
|   Loin Chop (1) | ½ lb. | 54 | 384 | 514 |
|   Rump Roast | ¼ lb. | 36 | 244 | 84 |

*Before cooking.*

| Fish | Portion | Sodium (mg.) | Potassium (mg.) | Calories |
|---|---|---|---|---|
| Clams (4 lg., 9 sm.) | 3½ oz. | 36 | 235 | 82 |
| Cod | 3½ oz. | 70 | 382 | 78 |
| Flounder or Sole | 3½ oz. | 56 | 366 | 68 |
| Lobster (1) | | | | |
|   Boiled, with 2 tbsp. butter | ¾ lb. | 210 | 180 | 308 |
| Oysters (5 to 8) | | | | |
|   Fresh | 3½ oz. | 73 | 121 | 66 |
|   Frozen | 3½ oz. | 380 | 210 | 66 |
| Salmon (pink, canned) | 3½ oz. | 387 | 361 | 141 |
| Sardines (8) | | | | |
|   Canned, in oil | 3½ oz. | 510 | 560 | 311 |
| Shrimp | 3½ oz. | 140 | 220 | 91 |
| Tuna | | | | |
|   Canned, in oil | 3½ oz. | 800 | 301 | 288 |
|   Canned, in water | 3½ oz. | 41 | 279 | 127 |

| Snacks | Portion | Sodium (mg.) | Potassium (mg.) | Calories |
|---|---|---|---|---|
| Candy | | | | |
| Chocolate Creams | 1 candy | 1 | 15 | 51 |
| Milk Chocolate | 1 oz. | 30 | 105 | 152 |
| Ice Cream | | | | |
| Chocolate | ½ pint | 75 | * | 300 |
| Vanilla | ½ pint | 82 | 210 | 290 |
| Nuts | | | | |
| Cashews (roasted) | 6-8 | 2 | 84 | 84 |
| Peanuts (roasted) | | | | |
| Salted | 1 tbsp. | 69 | 105 | 85 |
| Unsalted | 1 tbsp. | trace | 111 | 86 |
| Olives | | | | |
| Green | 2 medium | 312 | 7 | 15 |
| Ripe | 2 large | 150 | 5 | 37 |
| Potato Chips | 5 chips | 34 | 88 | 54 |
| Pretzels (3 ring) | 1 average | 87 | 7 | 12 |

| Dairy Products | Portion | Sodium (mg.) | Potassium (mg.) | Calories |
|---|---|---|---|---|
| Butter (salted) | 1 pat | 99 | 2 | 72 |
| Butter (unsalted) | 1 pat | 1 | 2 | 72 |
| Cheese | | | | |
| American, cheddar | 1 oz. | 197 | 23 | 112 |
| American, processed | 1 oz. | 318 | 22 | 107 |
| Cottage, creamed | 3½ oz. | 229 | 85 | 106 |
| Cream (heavy) | 1 tbsp. | 35 | 10 | 52 |
| Egg | 1 large | 66 | 70 | 88 |
| Milk (whole) | 8 oz. | 122 | 352 | 159 |
| Oleomargarine (salted) | 1 pat | 99 | 2 | 72 |

| Breads, Cereals, Etc. | Portion | Sodium (mg.) | Potassium (mg.) | Calories |
|---|---|---|---|---|
| Bread | | | | |
| Rye | 1 slice | 128 | 33 | 56 |
| White (enriched) | 1 slice | 117 | 20 | 62 |

| Breads,<br>Cereals, Etc. | Portion | Sodium<br>(mg.) | Potassium<br>(mg.) | Calories |
|---|---|---|---|---|
| Whole Wheat | 1 slice | 121 | 63 | 56 |
| Corn Flakes | 1 cup | 165 | 40 | 95 |
| Macaroni (enriched,<br>    cooked tender) | 1 cup | 1 | 85 | 151 |
| Noodles (enriched,<br>    cooked) | 1 cup | 3 | 70 | 200 |
| Oatmeal (cooked) | 1 cup | 1 | 130 | 148 |
| Rice (white, dry) | ¼ cup | 3 | 45 | 178 |
| Spaghetti (enriched,<br>    cooked tender) | 1 cup | 2 | 92 | 166 |
| Waffles (enriched) | 1 waffle | 356 | 109 | 209 |
| Wheat Germ | 3 tbsp. | 1 | 232 | 102 |

*Not available.

| Beverages | Portion | Sodium<br>(mg.) | Potassium<br>(mg.) | Calories |
|---|---|---|---|---|
| Apple Juice | 6 oz. | 2 | 187 | 87 |
| Beer | 8 oz. | 8 | 46 | 114 |
| Coca-Cola | 6 oz. | 2 | 88 | 78 |
| Coffee (brewed) | 1 cup | 3 | 149 | 5 |
| Cranberry Cocktail | 7 oz. | 2 | 20 | 130 |
| Ginger Ale | 8 oz. | 18 | 1 | 80 |
| Orange Juice | | | | |
| Canned | 8 oz. | 3 | 500 | 120 |
| Fresh | 8 oz. | 3 | 496 | 111 |
| Prune Juice | 6 oz. | 4 | 423 | 138 |
| Tea | 8 oz. | 2 | 21 | 2 |

| Fruits* | Portion | Sodium<br>(mg.) | Potassium<br>(mg.) | Calories |
|---|---|---|---|---|
| Apple | 1 medium | 1 | 165 | 87 |
| Apricot | | | | |
| Fresh | 2-3 | 1 | 281 | 51 |
| Canned (in syrup) | 3 halves | 1 | 234 | 86 |
| Dried | 17 halves | 26 | 979 | 260 |

| Fruits* | Portion | Sodium (mg.) | Potassium (mg.) | Calories |
|---|---|---|---|---|
| Banana | 1 6-in. | 1 | 370 | 85 |
| Blueberries | 1 cup | 1 | 81 | 62 |
| Cantaloupe | ¼ melon | 12 | 251 | 30 |
| Cherries | | | | |
| Fresh | ½ cup | 2 | 191 | 58 |
| Canned (in syrup) | ½ cup | 1 | 124 | 89 |
| Dates | | | | |
| Fresh | 10 medium | 1 | 648 | 274 |
| Dried (pitted) | 1 cup (6 oz.) | 2 | 1150 | 488 |
| Fruit Cocktail | ½ cup | 5 | 161 | 76 |
| Grapefruit | ½ medium | 1 | 135 | 41 |
| Grapes | 22 grapes | 3 | 158 | 69 |
| Orange | 1 small | 1 | 200 | 49 |
| Peaches | | | | |
| Fresh | 1 medium | 1 | 202 | 38 |
| Canned | 2 halves, 2 tbsp. syrup | 2 | 130 | 78 |
| Pears | | | | |
| Fresh | ½ pear | 2 | 130 | 61 |
| Canned | 2 halves, 2 tbsp. syrup | 1 | 84 | 76 |
| Pineapple | | | | |
| Fresh | ¾ cup | 1 | 146 | 52 |
| Canned | 1 slice and syrup | 1 | 96 | 74 |
| Plums | | | | |
| Fresh | 2 medium | 2 | 299 | 66 |
| Canned | 3 medium, 2 tbsp. syrup | 1 | 142 | 83 |
| Prunes | | | | |
| Dried | 10 large | 8 | 694 | 255 |
| Strawberries | 10 large | 1 | 164 | 37 |
| Watermelon | ½ cup | 1 | 100 | 26 |

*All portions weigh 3½ oz., unless otherwise noted.

| Vegetables* | Portion | Sodium (mg.) | Potassium (mg.) | Calories |
|---|---|---|---|---|
| Artichoke | | | | |
| Base and soft end of leaves | 1 large bud | 30 | 301 | 44 |
| Asparagus | | | | |
| Fresh | ⅔ cup | 1 | 183 | 20 |
| Canned | 6 spears | 271 | 191 | 21 |
| Beans, baked | ⅝ cup | 2 | 704 | 159 |
| Beans, green | | | | |
| Fresh | 1 cup | 5 | 189 | 31 |
| Canned | 1 cup | 295 | 109 | 30 |
| Beans, lima | | | | |
| Fresh | ⅝ cup | 1 | 422 | 111 |
| Canned | ½ cup | 271 | 255 | 110 |
| Frozen | ⅝ cup | 129 | 394 | 118 |
| Beets | | | | |
| Fresh | ½ cup | 36 | 172 | 27 |
| Canned | ½ cup | 196 | 138 | 31 |
| Broccoli | | | | |
| Fresh | ⅔ cup | 10 | 267 | 26 |
| Brussels Sprouts | 6-7 medium | 10 | 273 | 36 |
| Cabbage | | | | |
| Raw, shredded | 1 cup | 20 | 233 | 24 |
| Cooked | ⅗ cup | 14 | 163 | 20 |
| Carrots | | | | |
| Raw | 1 large | 47 | 341 | 42 |
| Cooked | ⅔ cup | 33 | 222 | 31 |
| Canned | ⅔ cup | 236 | 120 | 30 |
| Cauliflower | ⅞ cup | 9 | 206 | 22 |
| Celery | 1 outer, 3 inner stalks | 63 | 170 | 8 |
| Corn | | | | |
| Fresh | 1 medium ear | trace | 196 | 100 |
| Canned | ½ cup | 196 | 81 | 70 |
| Cucumber, pared | ½ medium | 3 | 80 | 7 |
| Lettuce, iceberg | 3½ oz. | 9 | 264 | 14 |
| Mushrooms (uncooked) | 10 sm., 4 lg. | 15 | 414 | 28 |

| Vegetables* | Portion | Sodium (mg.) | Potassium (mg.) | Calories |
|---|---|---|---|---|
| Onions (uncooked) | 1 medium | 10 | 157 | 38 |
| Peas | | | | |
| Fresh | ⅔ cup | 1 | 196 | 71 |
| Canned | ¾ cup | 236 | 96 | 88 |
| Frozen | 3½ oz. | 115 | 135 | 68 |
| Potatoes | | | | |
| Boiled (in skin) | 1 medium | 3 | 407 | 76 |
| French Fried | 10 pieces | 3 | 427 | 137 |
| Radishes | 10 small | 18 | 322 | 17 |
| Sauerkraut | ⅔ cup | 747 | 140 | 18 |
| Spinach | ½ cup | 45 | 291 | 21 |
| Tomatoes | | | | |
| Raw | 1 medium | 4 | 366 | 33 |
| Canned | ½ cup | 130 | 217 | 21 |
| Paste | 3½ oz. | 38 | 888 | 82 |

*Note: Because vegetable counts vary greatly from raw to cooked state, values are for cooked vegetables with no added salt unless otherwise noted. Frozen vegetables have virtually the same count as fresh vegetables, when cooked, unless otherwise noted.

A few extra moments in food selection and preparation can add years to your life by restoring a sparkling clean cardiovascular system and a healthy blood pressure.

# ELEVEN PRESSURE-RAISING COMPOUNDS TO AVOID FOR STRONGER ANTIOXIDANT POWER

Sodium compounds are chemical elements added to foods. As corrosives, they tend to erode your cells, grating against your exposed nerves, and forming dangerous clumps of free radicals. They also reduce or knock out the protective antioxidant power that you depend upon to have a healthy heart and blood pressure.

If this happens, your heart has to pump harder in a life-and-death battle to distribute blood throughout your body. The more fragments that become blockages, the harder your heart must pump. Up zooms your blood pressure. Down goes your antioxidant ability to dissolve and wash out these harmful molecular wastes.

To protect against this risk, you would do well to avoid these pressure-raising compounds. Remember, read labels before you use any product to see if it contains these destructive substances.

1. Salt (sodium chloride)—whether in cooking or at the table, it is destructive and should be avoided; this substance is also found in canning and processing.

2. Baking powder—used to leaven quick breads and cakes.

3. Baking soda (sodium bicarbonate)—use to leaven breads and cakes; sometimes added to cooking vegetables or used as an "alkalizer" for indigestion problems.

4. Brine (table salt and water)—used in processing foods to inhibit growth of bacteria; in cleaning or blanching fruits and vegetables; in freezing and canning certain foods; and for flavor as in corned beef, pickles, sauerkraut, french fries.

5. Disodium phosphate—present in some quick-cooking cereals and processed cheeses.

6. Monosodium glutamate (sold under various brand names for home use)—used in some packaged, canned, and frozen foods.

7. Sodium alginate—used in many chocolate milks and ice creams for smooth texture.

8. Sodium benzoate—used as a preservative in many condiments, such as relishes, sauces, and salad dressings.

9. Sodium hydroxide—used in food processing to soften and loosen skins of ripe olives, hominy, some fruits and vegetables. Also used in preparing Dutch process cocoa and chocolate.

10. Sodium propionate—used in pasteurized cheeses and some commercial breads and cakes to inhibit mold.

11. Sodium sulfite—used to bleach certain fruits for artificial color, such as maraschino cherries and glazed or crystallized fruit; also used as a preservative in some dried fruit. Read labels. *Tip:* select sun-dried fruits.

**Read Labels and Balance Your Blood Pressure.** If you must use packaged or prepared foods and beverages, read the labels. The presence of sodium in any form is your "red flag" to avoid the product. In so doing, you will be protecting your arterial walls against erosion. And you will also give "breathing space" to your antioxidants so they will build resistance to the threat of high blood pressure.

# HOW GARLIC IS A MIRACLE ANTIOXIDANT THAT REGULATES BLOOD PRESSURE ALMOST OVERNIGHT

Modern science has taken a clue from folk medicine in using garlic as a means of causing an antioxidant reaction that bolsters your resistance against the destructive effect of free radicals.

In particular, garlic causes an antioxidant process called *mitogenetic* reaction. This means garlic is able to stimulate cell growth and activity. This mitogenetic reaction helps in the process of synthesis or breakdown of lipids in the liver and prepares them for elimination, rather than storing them as broken fragments that could be threatening. Garlic uses this antioxidant reaction to help regulate your blood pressure almost immediately. It has an accelerated effect because of the force of the mitogenetic reaction.

## Lowers Blood Pressure within Two Days

Unable to plan meals properly, much-pressured construction engineer Nicholas C. was the victim of high blood pressure. He managed to cut down on salt and this did help bring down his readings to a slightly safer level. But he was still *not* out of danger. A visiting architect told him of a simple remedy he used that was given to him by a naturopathic physician that helped stabilize his pressure almost overnight. It was to use three to four cloves of garlic with a raw salad or even for a "snack" if the tangy taste could be tolerated.

Nicholas C. said that was preferable to blood pressure medications with their side effects. He started to eat garlic with his lunch and had his blood pressure checked two days later. The doctor was amazed. It was almost normal! Thanks to garlic, the antioxidant factor became activated almost immediately and stabilized his blood pressure within two days.

# ONIONS + GARLIC = FOREVER HEALTHY BLOOD PRESSURE

A combination of these two powerful antioxidant foods can work miracles in helping you achieve a "forever healthy" blood pressure. They appear to increase their antioxidant force when used together.

Onions are a prime source of antioxidants that zero in on *thromboxane,* a toxic free radical that could cause your blood pressure to soar. Onions use their antioxidants to guard against platelet aggregation, which can trigger off dangerously high blood pressure.

Garlic is a prime source of selenium (the valuable antioxidant that is needed to normalize blood pressure), and also prevents cellular adhesion and clot formation.

A *combination* of both of these antioxidant foods initiates a powerful buffering action from within that gives you natural immunity to the risk of high blood pressure.

Both onions and garlic release antioxidants that inhibit the treacherous buildup of wastes that could raise your blood pressure. Plan to use this combination on a daily basis for the sake of your pressure and your life.

# ALL-NATURAL ANTIOXIDANT HEALTH TONIC

If you turn up your nose at the volatile scent of onions and/or garlic, you can enjoy their benefits used as a tasty tonic.

In a glass of fresh vegetable juice (salt-free, please) place several slices of fresh onion and three or four garlic cloves.

Blenderize until frothy for just two or three minutes, then sip slowly. In this form, you will have a tangy and tasty treat that is not only a thirst quencher, but a powerful source of high biologically-acting antioxidants. Within moments, the selenium and allicin compounds will perform their therapeutic properties in building immunity to the risk of high blood pressure.

Just one glass a day of this "All Natural Antioxidant Health Tonic" and you may well be safe from cardiovascular distress.

## Reduces Pressure, Enjoys Healthy Reading in Three Days

Adelle K. went on a salt-free food program, but her blood pressure reading was still in the danger zone. Her diet therapist said she needed a strong buffer of antioxidants to help balance her pressure. She was told to use onions and garlic in her salads on a daily basis, but Adelle K. sneezed and sputtered from their volatile effects. She was advised to drink these vegetables as an "All-

Natural Antioxidant Health Tonic." Just one glass per day was all she needed. Adelle enjoyed it so much, that she had two glasses a day; she could feel improved health almost from the start. Three days later, when she had a pressure reading, the amazingly good news was that she was in the safe zone of 120/80. Thanks to this miracle tonic, she was saved from the risk of prolonged high blood pressure.

**Benefits of This Health Tonic.** The onion and garlic release antioxidants that fight off excessive platelet aggregation which can trigger off potentially dangerous clotting that is the forerunner of a heart attack or stroke.

These foods help keep control of serum cholesterol and triglycerides, which might otherwise clog your cardiovascular system and predispose to conditions of high blood pressure.

With this "All-Natural Antioxidant Health Tonic," you can drink your way to immunity from high blood pressure and related cardiovascular ailments.

## WHOLE GRAINS COUNTERATTACK PRESSURE RISE

Whole grains such as bran, wheat germ, oats, buckwheat, groats, and millet, are powerful antioxidants that can perform two valuable functions: (1) they help bring down excessive blood pressure; (2) they help keep it in a healthful balance.

Whole grains are prime sources of fiber, the substance that is able to push plasma cholesterol levels down, an important factor in blood pressure control. The same fiber is then able to release antioxidants that block absorption of many fatty elements and then break them down for easier elimination.

A bowl of hot oatmeal, for example, with some fruits cooked right in for natural flavor and sweetening is nourishing and also potent in keeping your pressure in check. It offers both fiber and pectin, a valuable antioxidant that protects against the risk of clots, which are always a threat for the hypertensive. Plan to have this cereal at least three times weekly for good antioxidant fortification, especially in the morning when you face your day's chores.

# HOW TO DOUBLE THE PROTECTIVE POWER OF ANTIOXIDANTS AND KEEP YOUR PRESSURE IN A HEALTHY BALANCE

Antioxidants may be considered the antidotes for blockages by free radical fragments that "choke" your arteries and predispose to high blood pressure. Boosting your intake of antioxidant foods such as garlic, onions, and whole grains, is a major step in the right direction. At the same time, keeping a check on salt consumption is also vital for the survival and vigor of antioxidants. But even if you boost your intake of antioxidant foods, you need to follow some basic guidelines to help them function properly. You do not want to weaken or destroy antioxidant power with improper foods or health habits. If you improve your lifestyle with these suggestions, you will help double and even triple the protective power of antioxidants.

1. Watch your weight. Keep it moderate. Do not allow yourself to go over your doctor-approved level.
2. Go easy on consumption of animal fats and high-cholesterol foods. During the process of metabolic combustion, rancidity occurs, which causes a form of oxidation that creates molecular fragments. Consumption of animal fats in excess seem to have this reaction. Moderation is the key.
3. Say "no" to smoking of any sort and avoid smoke-filled areas. Tobacco smoke is as destructive to antioxidants as air pollution, which should also be avoided.
4. Say "no" to alcohol of any sort. It, too, cancels out much of the protective benefits of the antioxidants.
5. Invigorate your antioxidants with regular exercise. You will be putting youthful power into these helpful nutrients if you keep fit. Just 30 minutes a day of a doctor-approved fitness program will boost the vigor of your antioxidants.

With this simple five-step plan, you will give your body's supply of antioxidants a supercharge of vigor to help give you immunity to hypertension, the "silent killer" that is like a time bomb ticking in your system! Don't set it off with antagonists of healthy living!

# RAW FOOD PLAN BOOSTS ANTIOXIDANT POWER

Because free radicals cause blockages that raise both systolic/diastolic pressure, your goal is to have a simple cleansing diet for just two days to give power to your antioxidants.

*Basic Program:* Select any two consecutive days of the week. During these days, eat only raw foods, and drink raw juices. Eat nothing cooked. Eat whatever fresh fruits and vegetables you desire, in any quantity, and drink their juices, too.

*Antioxidant Benefit:* Your digestive system is spared the effort of having to metabolize heavier foods. Your antioxidants are free to work solely upon raw foods, using the nutrients in them to help uproot and cast out the harmful free radicals. This will strengthen your cardiovascular system.

**Blood Pressure Levels Off.** Once the harmful radicals have been broken down and eliminated, thanks to the antioxidants, your blood moves more swiftly through your veins and your blood pressure levels off.

If you follow this "Two-Day Cleansing Diet" just once a month, in conjunction with the other outline programs, your antioxidants will reward you with a clean body and balanced blood pressure.

## Cuts Dangerous Blood Pressure in Half in Two Days

Saleswoman Betty W. experienced recurring headaches which brought her to the family practitioner for help. That's when she was given the jolting news of her exceedingly high blood pressure. An exam showed she had a dangerous 300/200 reading. She needed speedy help, lest the blockages cause bursting of a vital artery. She was told to follow the raw food "cleansing diet" and also follow other guidelines for boosting antioxidant power. Betty W. did as she was told. She also added garlic to all raw vegetable salads to further enhance her antioxidant supply. Within two days, her recurring headaches eased; the greatest news was a lowering of her blood pressure reading to 150/100. She was out of danger! It was a simple program, but it brought down the life-threatening high blood pressure, all in just two days.

With the use of antioxidants, you need not be one of the every six adults stricken by high blood pressure as statistics show. You have an opportunity to build immunity to excessive blood pressure and enjoy a longer and healthier life, as well.

## SUMMARY

1. A major cause of hypertension is that of mischief-causing free radicals in your system.
2. Avoid salt, so your antioxidants have full power to protect you.
3. Plan menus with the sodium-potassium-calorie charts in this chapter.
4. Avoid the eleven pressure-raising compounds to put more power into your antioxidants.
5. Nicholas C. was able to lower blood pressure within two days by using garlic, a miracle antioxidant.
6. Combine onions with garlic for double-barrelled antioxidant power for stabilizing your blood pressure.
7. Adelle K. had a healthy pressure reading in three days with the use of a tangy, tasty, "All-Natural Antioxidant Health Tonic."
8. Whole grains help counterattack unnatural blood pressure rise.
9. A five-step program helps improve your basic health and antioxidant vigor.
10. Betty W. lowered her dangerously high blood pressure by half within two days by following a simple raw food program that was brimming with antioxidants.

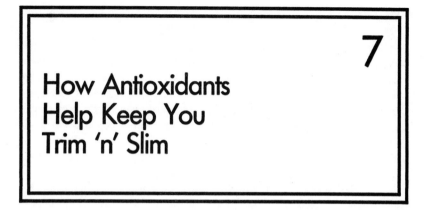

# How Antioxidants Help Keep You Trim 'n' Slim

**7**

A new and simple way of eating can offer you a youthful life by keeping you on the lean side. It can help you get rid of stubborn pounds and inches because it gets to the cause of your overweight; namely, a metabolic weakness that has allowed fatty wastes to accumulate in various parts of your body. Correct this defect with the use of antioxidants, and you will get rid of the fat right at its source. You will then have an opportunity to slim down with no need for torturous starvation diets that may cause nutritional deficiencies.

## THE "SETPOINT" REASON WHY MOST DIETS NEVER SEEM TO WORK

You have decided to follow a typical 1,000 calorie-a-day diet in the hopes that it will help bring down your weight and trim your waistline. Several weeks or months go by and you have lost some pounds, but you are still overweight and perhaps malnourished because of reduced portions and varieties of foods. What is wrong?

**Meet Your "Setpoint."** When your body is deprived of calories it once had, it assumes it is being "starved" and reacts by lowering its basal metabolism rate and activity level to compensate for the reduction in calories. As a result, you are able to sustain yourself on fewer calories without significant weight loss. Your body has a "setpoint" or particular level of fat that remains. Just as you have internal controls to keep your body temperature constant, you also have a thermostat for fat.

79

*Problem:* Cutting calories becomes a battle to overcome the "setpoint." Each time the fat level is reduced below your natural "setpoint," your body makes internal adjustments to resist the change and conserve body fat. One adjustment your body makes is to reduce the basal metabolic rate. (The amount of energy your body uses to run itself at rest.) When calories are reduced your body automatically adjusts to run itself on fewer calories. That is why you will find that your weight loss slows or even stops after a few weeks on a low-calorie diet.

*Solution:* You need to "reset" your "setpoint." You can do this by using antioxidants to help uproot and dislodge the accumulated fats that stubbornly cling to your cells. You need to "burn away" these fats. Antioxidants are able to overcome your "setpoint" by getting to the root cause and dislodging the fatty, free radicals that are responsible for your excess weight.

## HOW ANTIOXIDANTS HELP SLIM YOUR CELLS AND FLUSH OUT FATS

It is certainly wise to follow a calorie-reduced regimen coupled with exercise to help lose a certain amount of weight. But antioxidant foods and programs are needed to readjust your "setpoint" and begin a spontaneous combustion reaction that slims your cells and flushes out fats.

**The "Locked In" Fat.** The fat is stored primarily in the adipose cells (fat cells) in the adipose (fat) tissue. A fat cell is different in appearance from other cells. Most cells contain a large amount of cytoplasm, with the cell nucleus near the center of the cell. Fat constitutes almost the entire area of the adipose cell, and the cytoplasm and nucleus are displaced. Therefore, fatty radicals in the form of triglyceride, fill up the adipose cell. This is the source of your overweight—namely, the "locked in" fat. And if your "setpoint" is programmed so that you have much of this fat in your cells, the use of antioxidants will help make a necessary adjustment.

Putting it simply, the overweight person has a high "setpoint" and the lean person has a low "setpoint."

# ANTIOXIDANTS CORRECT METABOLIC SLUGGISHNESS

Your body has a control system—an inner thermostat for body fat—that seeks a constant set amount of fat in your body. Antioxidants are able to correct this "setpoint" and, in fact, lower it so that you can help get rid of this "locked in" fat and slim down. You have a variety of antioxidants to use to bring about this correction of metabolic sluggishness.

1. *Exercise.* A moderate amount of activity can accelerate your metabolism, lower you "setpoint," and even control your food cravings. Exercise causes the release of energy that is then converted to *adenosine triphosphate,* or ATP, a molecular compound composed of three phosphate groups. The phosphate bonds are high energy bonds that promote the burning of fats and the loss of pounds. Exercise is an antioxidant that will release fats from your cells, even as your "setpoint" is being lowered.

*Suggestion:* As little as 60 minutes of walking will burn up about 300 calories. Spend two hours a day on easy, but brisk walking, and this antioxidant exercise resets your "setpoint" so that you shed 600 calories; perhaps more. Bicycling at 5½ mph will shed 210 calories per hour. Swimming at ¼ mph will burn up 300 calories per hour. Enjoyable square dancing is an antioxidant activity that melts 350 calories per hour. Just set your goals and schedule a specific amount of exercise every day to keep your "setpoint" lowered and your weight melting away.

2. *Complex Carbohydrates.* These include starchy vegetables, whole grains, brown rice, legumes, peas. These are antioxidant foods that make it easy for you to lose weight. They exert an effect on the release of glucose in your bloodstream at a slow pace and over a long period of time; this helps your metabolism adjust your "setpoint" and burn up the fat that is locked in your adipose cells. Plan to eat a variety of these antioxidant complex carbohydrates daily. You will find the weight melting off with surprising ease.

3. *Fiber.* This is a non-nutritive substance because it is not digested in your system but provides bulk, a feeling of fullness, and a

natural appetite control. Fiber is a great antioxidant food that influences your *appestat,* the mechanism in your brain which controls hunger and satiety. Fiber sends a signal to your appestat that you are satisfied and this helps you eat smaller portions without hunger pangs. Fiber is found in whole grain bran, wheat germ, fruits, vegetables, seeds, nuts, and legumes. This antioxidant food has enormous bulk-forming capacity. It requires more chewing, which slows down the eating process, giving your brain enough time to realize that your body has eaten enough. This helps suppress your appetite.

*Benefit:* The antioxidant power of fiber attracts water, swelling up in your digestive tract to give you a sense of appetite satisfaction. Because fiber speeds up elimination of digested food, part of the fat may be excreted instead of absorbed and stored in your adipose tissues as girth-causing fat.

4. *Raw Fruit, Vegetable Juices.* Several glasses of fresh fruit or vegetable juices daily are able to maintain a steady weight loss. The antioxidants in the raw juices reduce serum triglyceride levels. They burn slowly, delicately releasing glucose (the important food for your brain) into your bloodstream so that you maintain an even level of blood sugar. These fresh juices help guard you against hypoglycemia or low blood sugar, the bane of many diets. Use them daily.

5. *Garlic.* This antioxidant food is a prime source of selenium (among other substances), which puts the brakes on the oxidizing free radicals that have entered your adipose cells and are to blame for your overweight. The antioxidants dispatched by garlic work with selenium to "trap" the fatty clumps, break them down, and prepare them for elimination. At the same time, garlic's antioxidants, such as selenium, help preserve the cell membrane and build resistance to fatty accumulation. In a sense, garlic helps your fat cells become immune to overload. It may be considered as an antioxidant that makes you immune to becoming overweight! Plan to have two or three garlic cloves daily, or more if your tastebuds can get away with it. But remember that the antioxidants in garlic protect you at the cellular level and this may well be the only way you can lose weight permanently.

With the use of these five antioxidants, you can adjust your "setpoint" and boost your basal metabolic rate and see the pounds and inches melt away.

## Loses 35 Pounds in 19 Days, Trims Waistline, Firms Up Sag, Looks Younger

Philip M. had a sagging body and a lifelong weight problem. His "setpoint" was at a level where he could not get rid of the excess poundage, no matter how he dieted or starved. So-called diet pills made him dizzy and so sleepy he could scarcely drive a mile without having the urge to doze off. They also caused blurred vision. He wanted to get rid of his weight and keep it off by using a natural method.

A physiotherapist diagnosed his case as having a sluggish metabolism. He was advised to try a simple antioxidant program to wake up his lax "setpoint." It called for one hour of walking every day. He was to omit refined foods and boost intake of complex carbohydrates and fiber. He was to give up caffeine beverages and switch to raw fruits and vegetable juices. He was to eat salads daily with several garlic cloves.

In just seven days, Philip M. saw his waistline becoming slimmer. His paunch began to flatten. His sagging body was becoming firmer. He had a more youthful look. Within 19 days on this antioxidant program he had lost 15 pounds and was the picture of slim health. The five antioxidant programs had readjusted his "setpoint" and cast out the accumulated fatty overload from his cells. He had won the battle of the bulge. On the antioxidant program, he could look forward to a new life of youthful slimness and health, too.

# HOW RAW FOODS CAN KEEP YOUR CELLS SLIM FOREVER

Fresh raw fruits, vegetables, seeds, nuts, and whole grains are powerhouses of high concentration of antioxidants. They work *within* your cells to uproot and dislodge the accumulated fats that are responsible for your overweight. In contrast, cooking foods tends to weaken, deactivate, or destroy some of the antioxidants. Canned, processed, frozen, dehydrated, precooked, and prepackaged foods have been subjected to temperature and chemical extremes which destroy these valuable fat-fighting antioxidants. Therefore, to give yourself a supply of adipocyte-slimming antioxidants, you need to partake of raw foods as often as possible.

**Cook Only if Food Requires It.** Obviously, you must cook beans, collards, and some other vegetables. Therefore, make it a rule to cook such foods but *only* if they cannot be eaten raw. True, you will deactivate or weaken antioxidants with this method, so make it another rule to gently steam such vegetables until tender enough for chewing and eating. Be sure to balance your food intake with lots of raw vegetables for super antioxidant cell-cleansing power.

## ANTIOXIDANTS IN RAW FOODS WASH AWAY CELL FAT OVERNIGHT

Some of the leading and most exclusive health spas of the world are able to stimulate dramatic weight loss in their top-paying clients by putting them on simple, but powerfully effective, raw food fasts. This type of program enables you to eat while antioxidants help wash away cell fat. A bonus here is that this antioxidant fat-scrubbing process works overnight while you sleep. You enjoy raw foods during the day; their powerful antioxidants work speedily in reducing your "setpoint" so that the cells are slimmed overnight. You can actually wake up much slimmer, thanks to this simple raw food program.

## CALORIE CONTROL = CELL CONTROL

Were you born to be fat? Based on the "setpoint" arrangement, this is a partial truth. Compare it to a home thermostat. You set the temperature at a certain level and while the room temperature varies around that level, it returns to it so that it fluctuates around this point at which you set the thermostat. Applying this example to yourself, you may be biologically programmed to weigh a certain amount. You may think you have a "built-in" weight regulatory system. And it has its beginning in your cells.

**The Fat Is in Your Cells.** Under the microscope your cells look like large bubbles; each cell has a single large droplet of fat. In some people, these droplets are enlarged much more than in others. You not only may have bigger cells storing more fat, but you may have more cells. Normally, a person may have 30 billion cells. But if you are always overweight, you may have five or ten times that amount of cells. And each one becomes overloaded with excessive amounts of fat that just do not melt away.

**Why You Gain Weight.** You may gain weight not because you eat more than others, but because your body is not burning off excess calories in the same way that lean people do. You have a weakness in your process of *adaptive thermogenesis;* that is, your body adapts so that there is less caloric burn-off than in other bodies. This is a biological defect that is in need of correction. This can be done by controlling calories, as a start, and by using antioxidants to help step up your basal metabolic rate. By stimulating your adaptive thermogenesis process, you will help burn up more accumulated stubborn fat from your cells.

**Calorie Control is the First Step.** If you have this sluggishness of your adaptive thermogenesis process, you need to be careful about your caloric intake. Basically, it takes 3,500 calories to add to one pound of fat. But something else happens. Any excess calories (even 100) will become transformed into fats that accumulate in your adipose tissues. This causes a condition called a *putative abnormality in neural functioning.*

**What Does This Mean?** The nerve cells become heavily laden with caloric fats. The unused calories (remember, only a few dozen are enough to cause mischief) have no where to go but to your adipose cells. There they cling together, especially on your nerve cells which attract them with sensitized magnetism. *Problem:* Nerve irritation leads to anxiety, causing overeating and more weight gain.

Therefore, to lower your "setpoint" and adjust your biological clock, do nature one better. Control your calories. This is the important initial step in getting rid of lifelong fat and being forever free of overweight.

## TEN STEPS TO BOOST CELL SLIMMING

1. Select fish, turkey, or chicken, which have fewer calories (less fat, too) than an equal size serving of red meat. Be sure to trim off all visible fat before cooking and before eating.
2. Drink skim or low-fat milk instead of whole milk.
3. Choose low-fat dairy products instead of creamed cheeses.
4. Bake, boil, stew, roast, or broil meat without adding fat.

5. Cook meat in fat-free vegetable bouillon.
6. Use fresh fruits instead of canned, frozen, or dehydrated types, or in cakes, pastries, and pies.
7. Avoid sugar. Read labels of any packaged foods you must use.
8. Avoid fried foods, creamed vegetables, creamed soups, extra sweet cereals, sweet desserts, and so forth. All are high in calories.
9. Carefully select the foods you eat (see chart on pages 86-90). Calories can add up quickly. One small baked potato yields about 100 calories; if that same potato is French fried, it yields nearly 400 weighty calories. If you consume the potato in the form of potato chips, it could give you nearly 650 calories per average portion. This is a dangerously high amount of fatty calories that can cause cellular engorgement and bloating.
10. Reduce the size of your portions.

With these basic guidelines, you should be able to control caloric intake, and improve your antioxidant powers to help you slim down much easier and swifter, too.

| Milk and Milk Products | Amount | Average Calories |
|---|---|---|
| Whole Milk | 8 oz. | 160 |
| Evaporated whole milk (undiluted) | 4 oz. | 170 |
| Evaporated skim milk (undiluted) | 4 oz. | 90 |
| Low fat milk (99% fat-free) | 8 oz. | 115 |
| Buttermilk | 8 oz. | 115 |
| Liquid skimmed milk | 8 oz. | 105 |
| Nonfat dry milk | ⅓ cup | 95 |
| Yogurt: Plain | 8 oz. | 135 |
| Vanilla & Coffee | 8 oz. | 200 |
| Fruit flavored | 8 oz. | 285 |
| Cheese: Hard (American, Swiss) | 1 oz. | 105 |
| Ricotta, partially skimmed | 1 oz. | 50 |
| Creamed cottage & farmer | 1 oz. | 40 |
| Pot or low fat cottage | 1 oz. | 20 |
| Egg | 1 large | 80 |

| Fish—Fresh or Frozen | Amount | Average Calories |
|---|---|---|
| Fat-mackerel, smelts | 1 oz. | 65 |
| Lean-cod, flounder, porgy, whiting | 1 oz. | 40 |
| Canned-tuna, salmon, sardines | 1 oz. | 55 |
| Shellfish-clams, oyster, shrimp, lobster | 1 oz. | 25 |

| Meats—Fresh or Frozen | Amount | Average Calories |
|---|---|---|
| Pork | 1 oz. | 90 |
| Ham, Beef, Lamb | 1 oz. | 80 |
| Veal, Chicken, Liver | 1 oz. | 65 |

**Luncheon Meats**

| | | |
|---|---|---|
| Frankfurter | 1 (2 oz.) | 170 |
| Bologna, Salami, Liverwurst | 1 oz. | 90 |
| Boiled Ham | 1 oz. | 70 |

**Dried Beans and Peas**

| | | |
|---|---|---|
| | ½ cup, cooked | 115 |

**Peanuts and Peanut Butter**

| | | |
|---|---|---|
| Peanuts | 1 oz. | 165 |
| Peanut Butter | 1 tbsp. | 95 |

**Bread, Cereals and Cereal Products**

| | | |
|---|---|---|
| Bread–all types | 1 slice | 65 |
| Rolls–Hard | 1 large | 155 |
| Hamburger, Frankfurter | 1 roll | 120 |
| Cereals–Cooked | ½ cup, cooked | 65 |
| Ready-to-eat | ½ cup | 55 |
| Muffins | 1 (2¾″ diam.) | 125 |
| Noodles, Rice | ½ cup, cooked | 105 |
| Spaghetti, Macaroni | ½ cup, cooked | 80 |

| Fruits | Amount | Average Calories |
|---|---|---|
| Orange | 1 medium | |
| Orange juice, unsweetened | ½ cup | |
| Grapefruit | ½ med. | |
| Grapefruit juice, unsweetened | ½ cup | 55 |
| Strawberries, unsweetened | 1 cup | |
| Tangerine | 1 med. | |
| Tomato juice | 1 cup | |
| Cantaloupe | ½ med. | |

**Berries**

| | | |
|---|---|---|
| Blackberries or Blueberries | ½ cup | 45 |

**Other Fresh Fruits**

| | | |
|---|---|---|
| Apple, Banana, Pear | 1 med. | |
| Peach | 2 med. | |
| Grapes, Cherries | ¼ lb. | |
| Pineapple | 1 cup | |
| Apricots | 4 | 80 |
| Plums | 3 | |
| Honeydew melon | ½ small | |
| Watermelon | Wedge 4″ × 6″ | |

**Canned Fruits—Syrup Packed**

| | | |
|---|---|---|
| | ½ cup | 100 |

**Dried Fruits—Uncooked or Cooked Unsweetened**

| | | |
|---|---|---|
| Apricots | 3 med. | |
| Prunes | 4 med. | |
| Raisins | 2 tbsp. | 65 |
| Figs | 1 large | |
| Dates | 3-4 | |

| Vegetables—Raw | Amount | Average Calories |
|---|---|---|
| Cabbage | ½ cup | 10 |
| Celery | 1 lg. stalk | 5 |
| Cucumber | ½ large | 15 |

| Vegetables—Raw | Amount | Average Calories |
|---|---|---|
| Escarole, lettuce Chicory | 1 cup | 10 |
| Radishes | 4 | 5 |
| Tomato | ½ med. | 20 |

| Vegetables—Cooked | Amount | Average Calories |
|---|---|---|
| Potato | 1 medium | 100 |
| Sweet potato | 1 medium | 165 |
| Corn, peas, Lima Beans | ½ cup | 75 |
| Dark green leafy | ½ cup | 20 |
| Deep yellow | ½ cup | 30 |
| Green | ½ cup | 15 |

| Soups | Amount | Average Calories |
|---|---|---|
| Bouillon | 1 cube | 10 |
| Broth, consomme | 1 cup | 30 |
| Clam chowder, Manhattan style | 1 cup | 80 |
| Tomato | | |
| Vegetable | 1 cup | 85 |
| Chicken Noodle | | |
| Split pea | 1 cup | 145 |

| Foods High in Calories | Amount | Average Calories |
|---|---|---|
| Fruit Pies | 4″ sector | 350 |
| Chiffon & Custard Pies | 4″ sector | 285 |
| Plain cake, iced | 3 oz. | 325 |
| Cup cake, iced | 2½ diam. | 130 |
| Angel Food cake | 2 oz. | 150 |
| Brownies | ⅔ oz. | 85 |
| Doughnut, sugared | 1 | 135 |
| Danish pastry | 3 oz. | 360 |
| Cookies | 1 lg. or 2 small | 100 |
| Crackers | 4 saltines | 50 |
| Bagel | 1 | 165 |

| Foods High in Calories | Amount | Average Calories |
|---|---|---|
| Matzoh | 1 square | 130 |
| Potato Chip | 1 oz. | 170 |
| Popcorn, sugar coated | 1 cup (1¼ oz.) | 135 |
| Pretzels | 1 oz. | 120 |
| Sugar, jam, jelly | 1 tbsp. | 50 |
| Gelatin dessert, plain | ½ cup | 70 |
| Chocolate pudding | ½ cup | 195 |
| Ice cream | ½ cup | 130 |
| Ice milk | ½ cup | 100 |
| Candy, chocolate | 1 oz. | 150 |
| Candy, hard | 1 oz. | 110 |
| Carbonated beverages with sugar | 12 oz. | 150 |
| Beer | 12 oz. | 170 |
| Wine, dry | 3½ fl. oz. | 85 |
| Wine, sweet | 3½ fl. oz. | 140 |
| Whiskey, gin, rum, vodka | 1½ fl. oz. | 110 |
| Cream cheese, heavy cream | 2 tbsp. (1 oz.) | 110 |
| Light cream | 2 tbsp. (1 oz.) | 90 |
| Sour cream | 2 tbsp. (1 oz.) | 50 |
| Butter or Margarine | 1 tbsp. | 100 |
| Oil | 1 tbsp. | 125 |
| French dressing | 1 tbsp. | 65 |
| Mayonnaise | 1 tbsp. | 100 |
| Bacon | 2 slices | 90 |
| Egg Roll | 1 portion | 300 |
| Chow Mein | 1 portion | 430 |
| Blintz | 1 | 200 |
| Knish | 1 | 480 |
| Pizza, cheese | 5½" sector | 185 |

# SIMPLE MEAL ADJUSTMENT TRIPLES SLIMMING ACTION

Eat your main meal at noontime and have a lighter meal at evening time. This simple adjustment can triple the antioxidant cell-slimming reaction.

**Activity Boosts Antioxidant Power.** If you habitually eat your major meal a few hours before bedtime, your antioxidant reactions have little opportunity to fulfill their maximum cell-slimming processes. When you are asleep, this activity is very slow, and the food can become stored as fat before you awaken.

Therefore, plan to eat your major meal in the middle of the day following it with physical activity (whether on the job, doing housework, or taking care of your usual responsibilities), then your "setpoint" lowers as activity boosts your metabolism and antioxidants are better able to help wash your adipose tissues, making weight loss more effective.

## Meal Changearound Creates Instant Cell Slimming

Arlene O. was embarrassed to purchase clothes at a local shop. She was constantly seeking larger and larger sizes. Weight just seemed to stick to her like glue, she lamented to the saleswoman who was half her size! The saleswoman told her of a simple diet change that had halved her own weight almost away. It was simple—just eat the high-calorie foods as early in the day as possible. Since energy is measured in calories, the adipose tissue becomes the caloric reservoir of the body. Physical activity that follows the main meal will boost the antioxidants to cause combustion of these calories. This will help slim down the adipose tissues.

Arlene O. made this change, with a caloric reduction at the same time. Almost immediately the weight started to vanish. Within 10 days, she had gone down to a size 10, and had enviable proportions. Arlene O. now could buy junior miss sizes . . . and she looked like a lovely junior, too, thanks to this instant cell-slimming reaction because of the simple meal changearound.

# HOW TO DRINK YOUR WAY
# TO YOUTHFUL SLIMNESS

Fresh raw fruit or vegetable juices are powerhouses of complex carbohydrates that rank high on the list of fat-slimming antioxidants. They also regulate fat metabolism. The antioxidants found in raw fruit or vegetable juices also initiate a protein-sparing action in your body; that is, they help divert the protein for cell growth and maintenance and guard against fatty overload.

Another important function of antioxidants in raw juices deals with fat metabolism. If there is a deficiency of antioxidants in your body, fats are metabolized too rapidly. Byproducts of fat metabolism, called *ketones,* are accumulated in the body. Unable to rid itself of the ketones fast enough, your body accumulates these toxic wastes and this could cause dehydration. Therefore, raw juices loaded with antioxidants serve to balance fat metabolism and protect against tissue overload and ketone toxicity.

The antioxidants in the juice work swiftly because they are almost instantly assimilated in this predigested form. Plan to drink fresh juices throughout the day as a means of giving your "setpoint" a boost and helping to guard against fatty overload in your tissues.

Following is a simple, but effective, weight-losing program that uses raw juices for antioxidant reaction in cell slimming.

*First Half of the Day:* Have several glasses of different fresh fruit juices, according to your taste. Be careful to drink two hours before or after your meal to avoid diluting eaten foods. Sip the juice slowly. Powerful complex carbohydrates and antioxidants will work swiftly to help lower your stubborn "setpoint" and create "cellular combustion" to help slim you down.

*Second Half of the Day:* Enjoy several glasses of different fresh vegetable juices. Their cell-scrubbing minerals are charged by the antioxidants in the complex carbohydrates to scrub away calories and fats that might otherwise lead to weighty accumulation.

Raw juices are powerhouses of antioxidants in the form of complex carbohydrates that get to the root cause of your overweight, namely, overloaded fat cells. By uprooting and dissolving this fatty overload, you will help correct the metabolic error that has caused a lifetime battle of the bulge for you.

Nature may have designated that you were born to be fat. At the same time, nature has provided antioxidants in foods, as well as in oxygen-producing exercise, to help counter this health risk. Use these methods and you not only will become youthfully slim, but will help yourself to live longer and healthier.

# TRIM POINTS

1. "Setpoint" is a biological reason why most diets do not work. Correct this stubborn internal thermostat with antioxidants and you will be able to get rid of excess pounds and inches.
2. Use the five antioxidants (these are found both in exercise and foods) to help correct metabolic sluggishness and lose excess weight swiftly.
3. Using antioxidants, Philip M. lost 15 pounds in 19 days.
4. Raw foods are powerhouses of fat-dissolving antioxidants.
5. Use antioxidants to stimulate your adaptive thermogenesis process, the reason for your overweight.
6. Control calories to accelerate weight loss with the ten step plan.
7. Arlene O. made a simple meal switch and lost weight quickly.
8. Fresh raw juices are super-powerhouses of antioxidants for burning up sluggish fat.

# Osteoporosis: How to Use Antioxidants to Protect Against "Aging" Bones

Osteoporosis can make you older before your time. It is a silent thief of youthful health because it has almost no symptoms. If allowed to progress, this condition can deteriorate the bone structure and cause premature aging, confinement and even eventual death.

## WHAT IS OSTEOPOROSIS?

It is a condition in which bone tissue decreases, causing the skeleton to be more susceptible to fractures. This reduction in bone mass progresses to such levels that osteoporotic (brittle) bones can no longer support the body. The bones slowly weaken, so slowly that the effects may not become evident until 30 or more years since the condition seized hold.

**Who Is the Victim?** An estimated 2 to 5 million people seek medical help each year for some problem linked to osteoporosis. Upwards of 15 million people have osteoporosis in some degree. The disorder is eight times more common in women than in men, partly because women have less bone mass to start with.

**Can Osteoporosis Strike Any Age Group?** This thinning of bone tissue is most common among post-menopausal women—one out of every four women over the age of 60 is affected by it; however, osteoporosis can develop in men and in younger women as well. Although the symptoms of osteoporosis are most visible in later years, the process that weakens bones actually begins 30 to 40 years before the first fracture occurs. After age 35, both men and women begin to lose

bone mass. As the bones become lighter and thinner, fractures can occur more easily and heal more slowly because the body is not able to
form new bone as easily as it once did.

**Why Do Older Women Become Victims?** As a woman
ages after menopause, her body's production of sex hormones,
including estrogen, declines. Estrogen seems to have a special
regulating influence on bone substance. This hormone is believed to
slow down the process of bone destruction. Estrogen also improves the
absorption of calcium by the intestine (that is, from food). With estrogen deficiency in women in their post-menopause years, osteoporosis is
more likely to occur.

**How Early Is the Risk?** Bone formation goes on until age 25.
In young adults, the skeleton is in a relatively steady state with bone
formation equaling bone resorption (bone loss). Bone loss begins earlier
in women than in men and speeds up after menopause. A combination
of low initial bone mass and early onset of bone loss in younger years
will lead to eventual osteoporosis.

**Can It Be Detected?** People with osteoporosis have no pain or
other symptoms until their bones become so weak that a sudden strain,
bump, or fall leads to a fracture. Often the condition is first discovered
on an x-ray taken for some other purpose. In younger years, it is
difficult for the thinning bone mass to show up on x-rays. There are
two highly sophisticated techniques that can measure the amount of
bone calcium in vertebral bone. The first is computer-assisted tomogra-
phy (CAT scan), and the second is the dual photon absorptiometry.
The CAT scan determines the amount or density of the bone in a single
lumbar vertebra. The dual photon absorptiometry measures the
amount of calcium in the total spine. These methods are a better diagnostic technique than x-rays which, for example, may not detect the
loss of 30 percent of the skeletal bone mass, a serious condition. It is
essential to have the skeleton examined early in life since bone loss progresses at about one percent a year from the early thirties.

**Can Osteoporosis Be Crippling? Fatal?** It can lead to dowager's hump, hip fractures, breakage of the spinal vertebrae, outward
curvature of the upper spine (kyphosis), a protruding abdomen because
the downward movement of the ribs forces the internal organs outward. There is often accompanying pain. Every year, 200,000

osteoporotic women over the age of 45 fracture one or more of their bones. Of these, over 40,000 die of complications following their injuries. Many of the remainder live altered lives because of chronic pain and disability. Osteoporosis is a major chronic condition and is the principal underlying cause of bone fractures in older people, especially women. A fall, blow, or lifting action, which would not bruise or strain the average person, can readily cause bones to break in someone with severe osteoporotic bones.

**Why Are Hip Fractures So Dangerous?** A person suffering a break in the upper part of the *femur* (long bone between the hip and knee) is many times more likely to develop a hip fracture of the opposite side. It is estimated that a hip fracture may reduce a woman's life expectancy by 12 percent. Thus, falls are the leading cause of accidental death in elderly women. Overall, hip fractures are the twelfth leading cause of death in America today.

Generally, some 6 million people are believed to have acute health problems related to weakened vertebra; as many as 8 million may have chronic spinal trouble. Wrist fractures also are extremely common among victims of osteoporosis; about 100,000 broken wrists are reported each year.

**Does Osteoporosis Have to Rob Your Youth?** For a long time it was thought that osteoporosis was an unavoidable consequence of aging. One could be young in every respect, except in his skeleton. This loss of bone mineral made people old before their time; it robbed them of their youth. Must you resign yourself to premature aging because of this condition? Not with the new knowledge of antioxidants, such as exercise and nutrients, that are able to strengthen your skeleton and give you a youthful skeletal structure no matter what your age.

## CALCIUM IS A BONE-STRENGTHENING ANTIOXIDANT MINERAL

Calcium is a valuable mineral that does wonders in protecting your skeleton against bone thinning or osteoporosis. The largest concentration of body calcium, approximately 99 percent is present in your skeleton, where this antioxidant aids in the development of strong and healthy bones and teeth.

Calcium serves other vital functions: it maintains normal heart rhythm, regulates nerve conduction, and aids in blood clotting. Calcium constantly circulates in the bloodstream at relatively steady levels. If not enough calcium is available from food sources, this mineral is siphoned off from your skeleton to enter the bloodstream. Over a period of time, this constant calcium drainage can lead to osteoporosis. (It is more common than arthritis, and three times more common than diabetes.) This need not happen, or at least it could be nipped in the bud, with the availability of adequate calcium.

**The Protective Power of Antioxidative Calcium.** Your bones may not be able to absorb as much calcium as required because of the interference by free radicals; these foreign substances will "steal" oxygen otherwise intended for segments of your bone mass. Oxygen is needed for calcium to be properly absorbed. When the free radicals use it up, "oxygen starvation" damages the cellular honeycomb membranes of your skeletal structure and this brings on osteoporosis.

Calcium offers an antioxidant reaction wherein it foils the free radicals' efforts to absorb needed oxygen; calcium also blocks the destruction of cell membranes by these foreign elements and assists in their eventual removal from your bone mass and other body parts.

Calcium further strengthens your bones by creating a unique antioxidant reaction; it establishes a regulating mechanism or a "calcium thermostat" that controls calcium levels and bone mass so that you are protected against osteoporosis.

## HOW TO BOOST YOUR INTAKE OF CALCIUM

A rule of thumb is to take between 1,000 to 1,500 milligrams of calcium per day. This amount should be taken by men and women in their late twenties or early thirties as a means of making certain that this bone-building antioxidant mineral will be available for protection against osteoporosis.

A major source of calcium is milk, either whole or skim, but since an average eight ounce glass contains only 288–296 milligrams, you would need to consume at least four to five glasses of milk *every single day*. This could cause bloating in some people, it could be undesirable to others. Many are unable to tolerate milk or dairy products, and so they have to pass up this source. You may consider the following sources of calcium:

# CALCIUM CONTENT IN SOME FOODS

| Food | Amount | Milligrams |
|------|--------|-----------|
| Whey, dried | 4 ounces | 646 |
| Sardines, canned | 3 ounces | 372 |
| Milk (skim) | 8 ounces | 296 |
| Milk (whole) | 8 ounces | 288 |
| Swiss cheese | 1 ounce | 262 |
| Half-and-half | 8 ounces | 261 |
| Yogurt | 8 ounces | 245 |
| Cheddar cheese | 1 ounce | 213 |
| Spinach (cooked) | 8 ounces | 212 |
| Processed cheese | 1 ounce | 198 |
| Salmon (pink) canned | 3 ounces | 167 |
| Broccoli (cooked) | 8 ounces | 136 |
| Cottage cheese | 1 ounce | 27 |

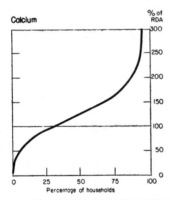

Calcium

%of RDA

Percentage of households

Calcium consumption levels of U.S. households. Note that 30% of the households were not consuming sufficient calcium—they were below the 100% of RDA. (From: *Nutrient Levels in Food Used for Households in the United States*, USDA, Science and Education Administration, January 1981)

**RECOMMENDED DAILY CALCIUM ALLOWANCES[1]**

| Group | Age (years) | Weight (lb) | (kg) | Height (in) | (cm) | Calcium (mg) |
|-------|-----|-----|-----|-----|-----|-----|
| Infants | 0-.5 | 13 | 6 | 24 | 60 | 360 |
| | .5-1.0 | 20 | 9 | 28 | 71 | 540 |
| Children | 1-3 | 29 | 13 | 35 | 90 | 800 |
| | 4-6 | 44 | 20 | 44 | 112 | 800 |
| | 7-10 | 62 | 28 | 52 | 132 | 800 |
| Males | 11-14 | 99 | 45 | 62 | 157 | 1,200 |
| | 15-18 | 145 | 66 | 69 | 176 | 1,200 |
| | 19-22 | 154 | 70 | 70 | 177 | 800 |
| | 23-50 | 154 | 70 | 70 | 178 | 800 |
| | 51+ | 154 | 70 | 70 | 178 | 800 |
| Females | 11-14 | 101 | 46 | 62 | 157 | 1,200 |
| | 15-18 | 120 | 55 | 64 | 163 | 1,200 |
| | 19-22 | 120 | 55 | 64 | 163 | 800 |
| | 23-50 | 120 | 55 | 64 | 163 | 800 |
| | 51+ | 120 | 55 | 64 | 163 | 800 |
| Pregnant | | | | | | + 400 |
| Lactating | | | | | | + 400 |

[1] *Recommended Dietary Allowances*, 9th ed., 1980, NRC-National Academy of Sciences, p. 186.

Note that the recommended daily allowances for calcium range from 360 mg to 1,200 mg. Note, too, that the allowances vary according to age, and that provision is made for added allowances for pregnant and lactating females.

*Suggestion:* A calcium supplement taken daily, with approval of your health practitioner, would be an excellent way of feeding your bones the all-important antioxidant mineral, calcium.

## VITAMIN D WORKS WITH CALCIUM TO STRENGTHEN BONES

Available primarily from the sun (produced by the ultraviolet irradiation of an inactive form of vitamin D in your skin), and in limited amounts from foods such as eggs, milk, and fish, vitamin D is stored in your liver in a partially activated form. It is transported to your kidneys where it is converted into its final, activated state. Vitamin D has an antioxidant reaction which conserves calcium in two steps.

1. It increases the absorption of calcium in the intestines.
2. It increases the reabsorption of calcium through the kidneys and is responsible for maintaining a proper level of the mineral in the blood.

**How to Boost Vitamin D Supplies.** Being in daylight for minimal amounts of time is helpful. You will also find vitamin D in certain foods. One small herring offers 330 units; a serving of salmon or tuna about 320 units; one medium egg offers 27 units. Three pats of butter gives about 28 units. One pint of whole, fresh milk gives you 200 units. You need about 400 units daily to put power into your calcium. Since this is a fat-soluble vitamin that is stored in your body, supplementation should be considered with the advice of your health practitioner. Consider natural fish liver oils as a good source of this important co-factor of calcium. And, of course, being out in the open air will help production of important vitamin D.

## FITNESS HELPS STRENGTHEN YOUR SKELETON

Keeping active is an important antioxidant way to strengthen your skeleton. The gentle pull on muscle tendons will stimulate bone formation. Inactivity can cause a loss of bone structure. The minerals just drain out of your bones when you are confined to bed for long periods of time or when you spend most of the day sitting. Fitness is an antioxidant way for maintaining healthy bones and avoiding osteoporosis.

**Helpful Antioxidant Exercises.** You will increase your bone mass by certain exercises that combine movement, pull, and stress on the long bones of your body. *Suggestion:* Try walking, jogging, bicycling, hiking, rowing, jumping rope. If performed with vigor, these activities become aerobic or antioxidant, which means that they tone your body and cause calcium to be deposited in your long bones. Just 30 minutes of any of these antioxidant exercises done on a daily basis will help strengthen your bone structure.

### Saved from Osteoporosis
### with Simple Antioxidant Program

Paula G. was diagnosed as having the beginnings of osteoporosis. She already walked with a stooped gait and felt her bones becoming fragile, even though she was in her early forties. She wanted to protect herself against a worsening of the condition. She took 1,500 milligrams of calcium daily, according to advice given by her dietician. She managed to get several hours of daylight to boost vitamin D production; she even took a tablespoon of cod liver oil daily. She spent at least 60 minutes a day doing one exercise or another. Within 20 days, another diagnosis showed she had halted the progression of osteoporosis. The physician who conducted the tests said she could make herself immune to osteoporosis with this three-step program: calcium, vitamin D, and exercise. They had begun the bone-saving antioxidant reaction of protecting against mineral loss.

## BEWARE OF THESE "BONE-ROBBERS"

The antioxidant power of nutrients and exercise will be blocked if you allow yourself to be subjected to these eight antagonists:

1. *Salt.* As salt is excreted, it tends to pick up calcium and take it out of your system. There is a relationship between salt and osteoporosis because of this process. Avoid salt and you may protect your calcium reserves.

2. *Coffee.* Whether it is the caffeine or other chemicals in it is not certain, but coffee appears to cause calcium loss from the bloodstream; it means that calcium is drained away from your bones to be used by your blood. It is best to avoid coffee in any form.

3. *Oxalates.* Compounds found in certain green vegetables such as asparagus, rhubarb, beet greens, spinach, sorrel, and dandelion greens. In your intestine, these oxalates combine with calcium to form large, insoluble complexes or free radicals that cannot be absorbed. While these are good foods, they should be eaten in moderation if you are suffering from osteoporosis.

4. *Phytates.* These are phosphorous-containing substances found largely in the outer husks of cereal grains, particularly bran and oatmeal. Phytates combine with calcium in the intestine and interfere with absorption. Again, whole grains are nourishing but if osteoporosis is a problem it is best to use them in moderation.

5. *Fiber.* It combines with intestinal calcium and creates free radicals that cannot be absorbed. While fiber is an essential item, the rule should again be moderation. You can obtain your fiber from fresh fruits, vegetables, and brown rice instead.

6. *Stress.* It decreases the absorption of calcium and causes much to be given off in waste. Stress automatically stimulates release of more adrenal hormones which can break down your bones. Stress also uses up a lot of calcium. Whether you suffer from emotional or physical stress, you should boost your intake of calcium. And, of course, try to avoid stress as much as possible for the sake of your bones and your general health, too.

7. *Antacids.* If they contain aluminum, they cause a negative calcium balance. Other chemicals may also block calcium absorption. Discuss proper medication with your health practitioner. Often, a happy medium is possible by boosting calcium supplementation, as prescribed.

8. *Smoking.* It definitely accelerates the loss of bone and is involved in the risk of osteoporosis. You would do well to kick the habit; at best, cutting down will also help reduce loss of nutrients. Tobacco smoke appears to create free radials that are corrosive and destructive to your bone mass.

Be on guard against the "bone-robbers" as part of your antioxidant plan to build resistance against osteoporosis.

## How Antioxidants Solved the Mystery of "Shrinking Bones"

Librarian Margaret N. started to lose height; she feared she was "shrinking" because of a mysterious ailment. Her physician said she was losing calcium from the osteoid matrix, or soft framework, at a dangerously high rate. Her ability to absorb calcium from food was weakened because she was in her mid-fifties. This further worsened the net bone loss. He recommended that she take a prescribed dosage of 1,500 milligrams of calcium daily. At the same time, he consulted her physical history and recommended that she give up salt, coffee, and smoking which were blocking absorption of the antioxidant mineral.

Margaret N. followed the program with some doubts; she had tried calcium supplements before, but because the "bone robbers" mentioned continued to do their damage, the program did not work. This time, however, by giving up salt, coffee, and smoking, the antioxidant effect of calcium worked swiftly. Within 12 days, she was diagnosed as having stronger bone mass. By the end of 26 days, Margaret N. had healthier bones and was protected against increasing osteoporosis. The half-inch of height she had lost because of bone mass shrinkage was not to be replaced but there would be no more losses, thanks to daily intake of the antioxidant calcium supplement.

# HOW TO "TIME CLOCK" MINERALS FOR MORE EFFECTIVE ANTIOXIDANT PROTECTION AGAINST OSTEOPOROSIS

When and how you take your calcium can have a decisive effect on protecting against the oxygen-devouring free radicals that can cause osteoporosis.

Calcium is best absorbed in small amounts. It is best to take supplements between meals with a small glass of milk or yogurt. Save about one-third of your daily dose for just before bedtime, since your body loses larger amounts of this important antioxidant when you sleep. *Reason:* When you are fasting or immobile, calcium is extracted from your bones. (All the more reason to include exercise as part of your plan to protect yourself against osteoporosis.)

**Eight Tasty Ways to Add Calcium to Your Food Program.** Be always on the alert for increasing your calcium intake in your diet. You can use any of these tasty methods to help promote this important mineral absorption in your system.

1. Prepare homemade soup by using stock from bones. Add a small amount of vinegar to dissolve the calcium out of the bones. As the stock boils, the calcium combines with the vinegar and erases the taste of the vinegar. To dispose of any vinegar odor, just remove the lid and let it boil off before adding vegetables.
2. Use the same vinegar method when cooking bone-containing meats. The vinegar tenderizes the meat and also shortens cooking time. Use leftover juices for gravy as they are top-notch sources of calcium.
3. Flavor vegetables with shredded or grated cheese, instead of butter. Parmesan cheese is great for adding flavor and calcium.
4. Garnish soups or salads with cheese cubes; or try tofu (a soybean product high in calcium) to boost nutritional value.
5. Select very deep green lettuce leaves as a base for salads; these offer calcium as well as vitamins and other minerals that work harmoniously to strengthen bones.
6. If you pickle fruits or vegetables, do so with calcium chloride as a replacement for sodium chloride (table salt).
7. Use powdered nonfat dry milk wherever it is possible. You can use it as a thickener in soups, casseroles, and sauces. Just one teaspoon gives you 50 milligrams of calcium that is *fat-free*.
8. Add about ¼ cup of the same powdered nonfat dry milk to baked goods such as bread, cakes, cookies, muffins. It boosts the calcium levels and you can eat your way to a stronger body, at any age!

Missing a step while walking down the stairs; getting a heel caught in a grate; falling because of an oil slick are all unfortunate causes of hip fractures, cracking of the spinal vertebrae, height loss, humped backs. There is no need to wait until these tragedies happen to know you have osteoporosis. Nip it in the bud. Begin as early as age 25, when one out of every ten women already has abnormally low calcium stores in her bones. In your middle or later years, follow the antioxidant bone-saving programs that have been outlined in this chapter to help protect you from disability. These programs will also help you stay young to enjoy a strong and healthy life in your later years.

# WRAP-UP

1. A silent condition, osteporosis has almost no symptoms as it takes the mass out of your bones to create a brittle and fracture-vulnerable skeleton. It afflicts over 15 million people a year and the figure is rising.
2. Calcium has antioxidant properties that strengthen your bones and protect against osteoporosis.
3. Check the list of calcium-containing foods and plan your diet accordingly.
4. Make certain you have enough vitamin D, because it works with calcium to create an antioxidant protection against brittle bones.
5. Fitness is a physiological response that helps nutrients become better absorbed for stronger bones. Select any of the specific antioxidant exercises.
6. Paula G. had dowager's hump and fragile bones; she was saved from serious osteoporosis by taking calcium and vitamin D daily.
7. Note the eight "bone-robbers" and avoid them for better immunity to osteoporosis.
8. Margaret N. used simple antioxidants to save herself from "shrinking bones."
9. Add calcium to your food program with the list of eight tasty tips.

# How to Banish the Blues and Brighten Your Lifestyle

Are you all tied up in knots? You can't stop worrying? Does stress make you edgy? Are your nerves ready to scream? Do you suffer from blue moods? You could be heading for an emotional collapse. You have built up an overload of negative byproducts within your system that are grating against your nerves, making you irritable, and giving you a sour disposition. You have to adjust your way of life with a better attitude and it can start with a correction of oxidation, the root cause of your so-called irritability.

## HOW TO DETERMINE IF YOU ARE UNDER STRESS

Before using various antioxidants to help banish the cause of the blues so that you can enjoy a more cheerful and rewarding lifestyle, it is helpful to identify your particular condition. You can do it with several very simple self-tests.

**Stress or Pressure?** You have endless chores to fulfill either at work or home (or both) and someone says you are under a lot of stress. Is it the same as pressure? Not exactly. It is important to differentiate between the two so that the proper antioxidants can be used to banish the blues. Pressure means having to do a lot of work, meeting responsibilities, carrying out obligations, and so forth. Most folks can cope with pressure because in overcoming it, it gives a feeling of pride and accomplishment. But stress can be nerve-grating. Are you a victim of it? Ask yourself these three questions:

105

1.  Are you in a situation which makes you feel helplessly trapped?
2.  Do you feel that you are about to lose control of the situation and yourself?
3.  Have you lost control and are seized with an inner sensation of helplessness?

If you have said yes to one or more of these questions, then you are a victim of stress and its inner pouring out of free radical byproducts that are chafing away at your nerves.

## CHECKLIST OF SYMPTOMS OF PROLONGED STRESS

Once your cells and tissues have become filled with the free radical byproducts of stress, the irritation persists. You may think you can control the situation by running away. But the molecular fragments are still in your body and the feeling of depression will persist until the antioxidants clear them out. To determine that this upheaval is taking place in your body, note these symptoms:

- Do you try to do two things at the same time?
- Do you eat fast and leave the table as soon as you have finished?
- Are you compulsive about being exactly on time?
- Do you find it difficult to sit quietly and do nothing?
- Are you being told by others to slow down?
- Do you blink or move your eyes rapidly while talking?
- Must you tap your fingers or jiggle your knees all the time?
- Do you interrupt or hurry up the speech of others?
- Do you sit on the edge of your chair as if poised for instant takeoff?
- Do you pound your fist for emphasis or talk with your hands?
- Do you make jerky movements and bump into or trip over things?
- Are you easily irritated if you have to wait for any reason?

If you have several or more of the preceding symptoms, then you may well be in the grip of an accumulated amount of irritants that are causing unrelieved stress. It can sour your disposition and take the joy out of life. It need not be this way. With the use of antioxidants, you can banish the blues and brighten your lifestyle with happy sunshine.

## BROWN RICE, WHOLE GRAINS, WHEAT GERM, AND BRAN ARE STRESS-MELTERS

During unrelieved stress, your adrenal glands react by releasing excessive amounts of *adrenalin,* a hormone that helps you cope with the problems that have you cornered. So far, so good. But your adrenals and related glands also release *catecholamines,* a group of substances that include norepinephrine and dopamine. These substances help meet the challenges facing you at the moment of stress. But when the situation is eased, and the adrenals stop production, these catecholamines do not entirely clear out of your body.

Fragments float around. They are the free radicals that cause oxidation. The cell membrane pits and corrodes and bacteria can enter all the more easily to cause irritation. Even after the stressful situation is over, these irritants remain to keep you feeling edgy and stressful.

**Whole Grains Are Antioxidants that Calm You Down.** The use of such whole grain products as brown rice, wheat germ, bran, and cereals will help counteract the corrosive effects of the free radicals and leftover wastes that are making you feel stressful. The whole grains are concentrated sources of B-complex vitamins, niacin, and pantothenic acid, which are able to knock out the biting vengeance of the leftover catecholamines and dilute their hydroxyl acid so that your cells are shielded from their burning reactions. You will soon calm down and feel much better in mind and body.

**Boost Your Whole Grain Intake.** The nutrients in whole grains are antioxidants and help brighten your moods, make you feel more stable, soothe your nerves. If you know you are facing unrelieved stress, or if you feel you are in the throes of such pressure that you are at nerve's end, you can find speedy relaxation by boosting your intake of whole grains. For example, breakfast could include a whole grain cereal with bran and fresh fruit slices; lunch could call for a double decker vegetable salad with sprouts on whole grain bread and brown rice pudding; dinner could be assorted seeds and nuts, vegetable soup or chowder with several tablespoons of wheat germ and/or bran. On this simple and tasty program, you can brighten your moods as the antioxidants in the whole grain dispose of the irritating byproducts—the free radicals that are clinging to your nerves.

### Laughs More, Enjoys Life on Whole Grain Plan

Oscar H. felt trapped. Endless responsibilities and deadlines made him feel like screaming. He snapped at his wife and youngsters and was just unable to get along with anyone. It was not like Oscar H. to be so irascible. He was the victim of radical fragments that were grating against his nerves. A nutritionist in his company's medical facility suggested that he correct the oxidant reaction that was responsible for his irritation.

Oscar H. was told to boost his daily intake of whole grains; he should also have rice bran, nuts and seeds, and also brewer's yeast because they were powerhouses of antioxidants that would nullify the leftover byproducts of his adrenal gland secretions. Oscar H. made this easy adjustment. He consumed whole grains daily in one form or another. Within three days, he felt calmer. At the end of six days, he was smiling and cheerful again. He felt like a new person. He coped with his daily deadlines and pressures because he was free of internal irritation, thanks to the antioxidant action of whole grain foods.

## THE ANTIOXIDANT MINERAL THAT MAKES YOU SMILE ALL OVER

Feel the blues coming on? Is everything getting the best of you? Are you troubled with bouts of depression? They are all reactions to accumulated stress-causing free radicals. Your personality can be upset because of this nerve-grating by the molecular fragments. To help correct this disorder you need to boost your intake of magnesium, a soothing and attitude-brightening antioxidant mineral.

**Adjusts Your Attitude, Makes You Cooperative.** Magnesium is able to wash away fragments to cleanse your nervous system and relieve irritation. It adjusts the route of nerve conduction; it creates an antioxidant improvement in transmission at your myo-neuro junction where fragments could be especially irritating. It further improves muscular contraction so that you can function with a more positive attitude and open mind. Magnesium is a soothing, mind-improving antioxidant mineral.

**Cheer-Up Health Tonic.** Combine eight ounces of fresh vegetable juice with an assortment of nuts and seeds, a spoon of desiccated liver granules (available from a health food store) and blenderize for two or three minutes. Drink it slowly. Within moments, the magnesium in the nuts and seeds join with the B-complex and highly concentrated magnesium of the liver to uproot and discharge the accumulated free radicals so that your cells become calm and relaxed. The antioxidant power of this "Cheer-Up Health Tonic" works so swiftly, you will feel like smiling within a matter of moments. This is the power of magnesium helping to brighten your mood.

## From "Rough Mood" to "Happy Talk" in Four Hours

Managing a household and a part-time job, not to mention long commuting hours, certainly put Louise Y. through the wringer. She was fit to be tied. She would snap loudly upon the slightest provocation. Living with her was like walking a tightrope! One false move and a shouting outburst would erupt.

Desperate to correct her "rough mood," she sought help from an orthomolecular physician who diagnosed her condition as an oxidative fallout, so to speak. It was grating on her nerves. She was told to boost her intake of magnesium. She tried the "Cheer-Up Health Tonic" early the next morning. Within four hours, she was bright and cheerful and bursting with "happy talk."

Louise Y. had counteracted the corrosive effects of oxidation with the use of this soothing mineral. Now she was happy again, thanks to the antioxidant power of magnesium in the "Cheer-Up Health Tonic."

# HOW CHEDDAR CHEESE CALMS YOUR NERVES

Can't unwind? The reason could be a blockage in your central nervous system. You need to get the clogged byproducts of combustion out of your system. Many of your cells and molecules become eroded by these peroxides that break down your immunity to stress and other external conditions. To help calm your nerves and cast out these free radicals, you need only have a small piece or two of cheddar cheese.

*Benefit:* This cheese is a richly concentrated source of *tryptophane,* an essential amino acid which is speedily converted into *serotonin.* This is a neurotransmitter that is able to stamp out the abrasive reactions of free radicals and caustic end-products and help you unwind. The response will be felt almost at once. Whenever you feel uptight, just loosen up with some cheddar cheese. Add whole grain crackers (no salt, please!) for soothing B-complex vitamins and you will be free of nervousness.

### Snack Foods Help Improve Mood

Mood swings made Brian G. feel like laughing and then shouting almost within minutes. He was faced with endless responsibilities and always said he loved to keep active, so he was at a loss as how to cope with these antisocial moods. He lost many friends and alienated members of his own family, too.

He was becoming irritated because environmental oxidants were eating away at his nerve cells. He sought help from a neurologist who suggested he counteract the irritating bite of oxidants by boosting his internal supply of serotonin. He was told to use snack foods. Yes, he could snack his way to cheerfulness! He was to use cheddar cheese, whole grain crackers, and seeds and nuts. He was not to take salt or sugar in any form. Munching on these foods throughout the day was the prescription.

Brian G. began to snack in the early morning and in the afternoon. Almost at once, his moods stabilized. He felt more at peace with the world around him. He hardly snapped at anyone and he was cheerful. He was a joy to live and work with. The snack foods, especially the cheddar cheese, had released serotonin as an antidote to the oxidants that were the cause of his irritation. Now he widened his circle of friends with his happy smile and cheerful disposition.

## THE ANTIOXIDANT THAT MELTS ANXIETY WITHIN MINUTES

Tensions, apprehensions, and irritability may have an oxidant cause, namely the presence of *lactate* in excessively high levels. (Lactate is a metabolic product created when you are subjected to intense activity of either body or mind.)

*Symptoms:* An excess of lactate (lactic acid) causes increasing symptoms of anxiety such as feelings of impending doom, fears of heart attacks, choking or smothering sensations, improper breathing, nervousness, tension and other excessive fears.

**Antioxidant That Melts Stress.** The mineral, calcium, can help dilute and negate the erosion caused by lactic acid upon your nervous system. Calcium is an antioxidant that neutralizes the stress-provoking reactions of lactic acid. Calcium reacts biologically with lactate, forming calcium lactate, and thereby binds lactate into a physiologically inactive form and reduces its capacity to produce anxiety.

As an antioxidant, calcium inhibits lactate's burning punishment on the nervous system. A clue to its behavior is in its antioxidant role in nerve impulse transmissions. Stated simply, calcium ions reside at the ends of nerve cells (termed synapses) and maintain electrical connections and communications between nerve cells.

In a stress-free nervous system, calcium combines with lactic acid around the sensitive nerve endings, creating an antioxidant reaction to block the acid from irritating your nervous system.

But if you have too much lactic acid, or a deficiency of calcium needed to perform the antioxidant neutralization, then you become fit to be tied. You may experience palpitations, tightness and lumps in your throat, and apprehension. This is the end-result of an excess of lactic acid. Calcium increase will soothe your nervous system and help you feel glad all over.

**Where Does Lactic Acid Come From?** It is a byproduct of glucose metabolism. When you are stressed (in body and/or mind), your body cells metabolize the glucose to produce energy without using oxygen. This process is termed *glycolysis.* The end-product of glycolysis is lactate. A buildup leads to fatigue and subsequent anxiety and muscle tension. You feel that you are caught in the grip of vise-like tension and just cannot relax.

**How to Use Calcium as an Antioxidant.** Calcium is available in dairy products as well as in supplements to be used with guidance by your health practitioner. If you consume at least 1,000 milligrams of calcium daily, you will help dilute the nerve-burning punishment of irritating lactate and you will soon feel cool, calm, and collected. It is as simple as that! A glass of milk (whole or skim contains approximately the same amount of calcium), a platter of cheese (salt-free, please!), and yogurt are just some of the sources of calcium, the antioxidant that helps you relax and enjoy life.

## Uses Cheese as a Natural Tranquilizer

Unrelieved pressures became a heavy burden for Dorothy X. There were times when she felt she just could not go on. Community responsibilities, raising a large family, and attending evening classes at a local college all made her irritable and tense.

Dorothy X. felt like exploding at times, and would snap back upon the slightest provocation. She resisted a suggestion that she try a prescribed tranquilizer because she was afraid of side effects and the risk of addiction. Instead, she asked an internist for a more natural approach. A diagnosis was made. She had an excess of lactate, a free radical waste that was causing her nerve irritation.

To wash out and neutralize this irritant, she was told to eat salt-free cheese. A prime source of concentrated calcium, this cheese would cause a valuable, mind-soothing antioxidant reaction. Dorothy X. would have a variety of cheeses on a daily basis; along with fresh fruit and whole grain crackers, they gave her the nutrient power she needed to counteract the effects of lactate. Within six days, she felt naturally calm. Dorothy X. no longer was jumpy; she had control over her emotions. She felt at peace with herself and her surroundings. She took additional evening courses and soon graduated at the top of her class. She was voted "the happiest student in the school!" Cheese, with the antioxidant power of calcium, had made her emotionally strong and healthy!

# HOW ANTIOXIDANTS COOL OFF YOUR STRESSFUL "HOT REACTIONS"

Since each person is different, levels of coping with everyday responsibilities are also different. For some people, the demands of work and an active family life can often cause more stress than their bodies can handle. They may have fallen victim to "hot reactions" or overresponding physiologically when under stress.

*Symptoms:* Your blood pressure rises sharply; the output of your heart increases; blood vessels become more resistant to blood flow.

Your heart must pump harder against greater resistance, as if trying to drive at top speed with the brakes on. A "hot reaction" deposits a flood of fragmentary molecules that could so upset your cardiovascular system, you run the risk of unexpected cardiac fatality. These dangerous free radicals create lesions in your nervous system called *contraction bands* which are related to the outpouring of catecholamines, those irritants produced by the adrenal glands. This happens during unrelieved stress which creates the "hot reaction" process that can be very damaging and threatening to your life.

*Antioxidant Solution:* Calcium, desiccated liver, and brewer's yeast are sources of antioxidants that are able to regulate your internal "hot reaction" so that it is less volatile. The antioxidants help knock out the irritating free radicals that cause an increase in such reactions. These antioxidant foods create internal immunity by preventing oxidation of the cell membrane. This extends its life (and your life, too) and helps damaged cells repair their chromosomes to guard against malignancy. In effect, these antioxidant foods can become natural tranquilizers.

**How to Use the Antioxidant Foods.** Plan to have some calcium daily, either from dairy products or from a supplement. Use one to two tablespoons of desiccated liver in a blenderized vegetable juice or in a casserole, soup, or stew on a daily basis. And a half to one teaspoon daily of brewer's yeast mixed in any vegetable juice or in baked goods will also provide the valuable antioxidants you need to cool off the "hot reaction" that is making life so tumultuous for you.

## EASY WAYS TO HELP YOURSELF GUARD AGAINST STRESS

Give antioxidants an opportunity to protect you against the dangers of stress. Change your attitude toward daily activities. A new approach will be helpful. Some suggestions are:

- Do something nice and unpredictable for a person very close to you.
- Smile at people in your home, workplace, street, store, and elsewhere.
- Every day, take 15 to 30 minutes alone and do nothing except listen to music that is soothing to you.

- Show an interest in others in your family or at work.
- Listen carefully to whatever someone is saying without diverting your thoughts and remain attentively silent until they have finished.
- Decide that minor errors need to be forgotten instead of continually worrying about them.
- Laugh at yourself!
- Periodically, take a look at yourself in the mirror no matter where you are and check to see if your face shows signs of irritation. Resolve to smile your way through any dilemma.
- Write or telephone or visit an old friend.
- Indulge yourself in simple pleasures and plan brief escapes to help yourself relax.
- Daydream! It's a great way to refresh yourself.
- Organize your day so everything gets done without panicking against self-imposed deadlines.
- If you must be with people who stir your anger, use your good sense of humor and keep reminding yourself (and others, too!) that life is here to enjoy, not to annoy.
- If you must make changes, do not attempt too many at one time.
- Reduce your time pressure by taking more rest stops to help ease your fear that time is running out.
- When dealing with others, make eye contact.
- If you find yourself in an uptight situation, politely explain, "I'm feeling upset now; I'd like to return a little later and talk further with you."
- Learn when you need to come to a stop; a brief retreat can be very soothing.
- It is very important to have someone to talk to, someone who understands your situation, and who will listen while you talk.

Stress is very much a part of modern life. Your objective is not to get rid of it, since this would not be at all possible. Instead, strengthen your reserves to resist the ravages of stress. You want to build immunity to the attending health risks of corrosive substances that can give you undesirable mood swings. With the use of antioxidants, you can banish the blues and brighten up your whole lifestyle.

# BRIGHT SPOTS

1. Take the simple home test that tells you whether you are a victim of prolonged stress.
2. Use whole grains as natural stress-melters that use antioxidant power to defuse irritating catecholamines.
3. Oscar H. brightened up his irritable personality with the use of whole grains as a source of soothing antioxidants.
4. For speedy tension relief, enjoy the "Cheer-Up Health Tonic." It works in minutes because of the high magnesium content.
5. Louise Y. went from a "rough mood" to "happy talk" in four hours with the antioxidant "Cheer-Up Health Tonic."
6. Brian G. used snack foods such as cheddar cheese to calm his nervous disorders.
7. Calcium is an antioxidant that melts anxiety which is traced to an excess of lactate, within minutes.
8. Dorothy X. used cheese as a natural tranquilizer.
9. Use the described antioxidants to help cool off your "hot reactions" that are causing stress.
10. Adjust your attitude toward daily responsibilities with the list of suggested new approaches.

# Wake Up and Enjoy Youthful Energy with New Molecules

Are you troubled with midday slump or early fatigue? Do you feel tired all the time? Is it a struggle to get out of bed in the morning? Are the days getting longer and longer because your mind and body are always exhausted? Then you may have a problem with low blood sugar or *hypoglycemia*. This means your cells and molecules have become over-burdened with free radicals from sugar sources that are causing "cross-linkage," that is, the binding together of large molecules and neurotransmitters that cause the stiffness and brittleness you feel as constant fatigue. An excess of the free radicals that clutter up your cells can cause this condition of hypoglycemia, recognized as constant ex-haustion, even in the early morning when you've had a good night's sleep.

## MOLECULAR OVERLOAD = HYPOGLYCEMIA

When you allow your molecules, especially your network of neurotransmitters, to become overloaded with oxidants or waste prod-ucts, you run the risk of having your energy sapped to the extent that you endure bouts of exhaustion because of hypoglycemia.

**Neurotransmitters Produce Energy.** Neurotransmitters are chemical substances released from nerve endings that transmit en-ergy impulses from one nerve to another. These neurotransmitters need to be kept clean and free of the corrosive effects of oxidants in order to help give you healthy and vigorous energy levels. In effect, they are molecules that store energy and must have free access to your network of cells, which are in constant need of charging. Yet, if you allow your molecules to become overloaded with oxidants, the result can be a reduced amount of energy and the so-called feeling of chronic fatigue.

**Hypoglycemia Causes Energy Loss.** Hypoglycemia means low blood sugar. Translated into simple lay terms, *hypo* means "low" and *glycemia* means "sugar." It may be considered the opposite of hyperglycemia or high blood sugar as seen in diabetes. When your molecules are subjected to a condition of low blood sugar, your metabolic functions go away and you start to feel a decline in energy. And more often, you run the risk of premature aging. You may feel depressed, irritable, suffer from headaches, tremors, tachycardia (palpitation of heart), muscle pain, and backache, forgetfulness, nervousness, moodiness, ringing in the ears, breathlessness, yawning, vertigo, and excessive sweating. These are often seen in folks in their middle years and are considered signs of "old age." Yet, a correction in hypoglycemia can erase these symptoms and bring about a feeling of rejuvenation and healthy vitality. It can be that simple!

The goal is to use antioxidants in specific foods as well as an easy-to-follow food program so that your molecules will be able to function harmoniously with your neurotransmitters to send forth a steady supply of youthful vitality.

## WHY DOES HYPOGLYCEMIA OCCUR?

Sugar stimulates your pancreas gland to secrete *insulin,* a hormone that helps transform the sugar and other substances into usable glucose, an important source of energy in your body and the *only* source of energy for your brain.

Too much sugar triggers off an overproduction of insulin. This burns up not only the sugar you have just eaten, but much of your reserves of blood sugar. Result: too little glucose in your blood. You now have physical reactions but also psychological symptoms such as lethargy, foggy thinking, depression, confusion, anxiety. Some people faint or their hearts thump so violently, they feared they were having a heart attack! Remember, your brain depends *solely* upon glucose for energy. Deprive it of this source, and it becomes erratic and malfunctioning. So we see that hypoglycemia happens when you have too much sugar that is burned up too quickly.

**Is Sugar the Solution?** It would seem very easy to just eat sugar to raise the levels in the bloodstream. But this gives you a rush of

# 118 *Wake Up and Enjoy Youthful Energy with New Molecules*

energy and a so-called "pick-me-up" that has a see-saw effect. You have a burst of vitality, but then you have a plunging letdown. It is this up-and-down reaction caused by sugar that makes it a "no-no" for those who seek stabilized energy.

**The "Yo-Yo" Reaction of Sugar.** Refined sugar, either as part of a snack or in a meal, causes a rush of energy. This is a short-lived boost. The pancreas, overstimulated by the influx of sugar, releases excessive amounts of insulin. Too much sugar is drawn from your blood. You feel this reaction as your physical and mental energies plunge downward. You experience fatigue, tension, nervousness, and disorientation. You have the "yo-yo" reaction of upward energy and downward fatigue. More sugar is definitely not the answer to hypoglycemia.

# LOW BLOOD SUGAR—DO YOU HAVE IT?

You can find out by having a glucose tolerance test, or GTT, as it is referred to in medical terminology. Your health specialist will ask you to prepare for the six-hour GTT. Assuming the test is done in the morning, you are told not to eat anything after last night's dinner. Absolutely no food at all after 10:00 or 11:00 P.M.

At the doctor's office, your first blood test is taken to determine your *fasting* blood sugar level. After that, you are given a glucose solution to drink. An hour later, another blood sample is taken. Five more samples are taken each hour; each sample is diagnosed for its blood sugar level.

If you are healthy, your sugar level rises to a figure such as 120. (A normal range is considered to be between 80–120 milligrams per 100 milliliters of blood.) Then the sugar should return to the fasting level before the test.

If you have low blood sugar, the natural rise is followed by a rapid drop below the normal fasting range. The *lower* and the *faster* it drops, the more severe the condition.

It is customary to take a urine specimen at the same time a blood sample is taken. Excess sugar is often spilled into the urine, particularly with diabetics. Because hypoglycemia can often be confused with diabetes and because a patient may have both conditions intermittently, it is valuable as a diagnostic adjunct to have a urinalysis with the blood test.

**How to Read Tests.** It is important for your health specialist to "read the curve" of your tests. That is, there are no set number or points which identify hypoglycemia with exactness. Some people walk around with it symptom-free. Others have neurotic or psychotic behavior on an almost similar glucose tolerance test reading. The test should tell not only how low the level drops, but how rapid the drop is. Also, the speed at which the glucose level returns to normal and how long it remains at the low point, are vital factors for your health specialist to consider.

*Example:* The curve drops to 50, but recovers to its pre-fasting level very swiftly, which indicates a mild case without noticeable symptoms. But—if it drops to 65 and remains there for several hours, such an extended low level may erupt in severe reactions.

Each person shows a different, individual curve, and is as personal as one's own fingerprints. The GTT should be used in combination with a clinical examination and a thorough case history and symptoms of the patient. Then a proper diagnosis can be made to fit your specific needs. "Reading the curve" is an essential part of the entire treatment.

## 15 ANTIOXIDANT STEPS TO MOLECULAR REJUVENATION AND YOUTHFUL HEALTH

You can correct the sharp fluctuations in blood glucose levels and guard against oxidants deposited by sugar by using molecular regeneration programs you can follow right at home. Each of the following 15 antioxidant steps are designed to undo the damage caused by cross-linkage of your molecules. The influx of sugar in any form deposits mutagenic, biologically destructive free radicals in your cells. The DNA–RNA genetic code becomes injured, perhaps incapacitated. This causes oxidative reactions that lead to glucose insulin imbalance, upset your blood sugar levels, and cause chronic fatigue and mental unrest.

The antioxidant steps that follow are aimed at rebuilding your genetic blueprint, erasing any interference by free radicals and restoring health and vitality to your DNA–RNA codes. They help undo the handcuff-like cross-linkage of your molecules and let them function freely and healthfully. In effect, you develop immunity to the destructive effects of the free radicals. Follow these steps (they're amazingly simple and astonishingly effective in just a short while) and rebuild your capacity for youthful energy, thanks to their antioxidant reaction and free radical cleansing power.

1. *Avoid All Forms of White Sugar.* This includes ice cream, pastries, cookies, soft drinks, candies, cakes and everything else that has white sugar in any form whatsoever.

2. *Avoid All Forms of White Flour.* This includes any commercially available bread (even though labeled brown or whole-grain). These may contain white flour which causes cellular clogging and deposition of the free radical wastes. Be cautious about packaged breakfast cereals, pastries, pies, gravies, etc. Read labels, or better yet, bake items yourself.

3. *Avoid Sugar-Free Soft Drinks.* Your molecules are abused not only by sugar, but by synthetic sweeteners that can cause deterioration and premature aging. Artificial sweeteners and flavorings, citric, phosphoric, and other strong acids that provide a fake sweet flavor are as harmful as the sugar they replace.

4. *Avoid Any Caffeine Product.* Caffeine whips up your energy levels, but then gives you a drop. Furthermore, this drug reacts corrosively upon your molecules and can cause internal deterioration. Whether in coffee, soft drinks, candies (many chocolates have caffeine), or packaged products, caffeine should be avoided for the health of your molecules.

5. *Avoid Any Form of Alcohol.* By drinking alcohol, you can burn off the filaments and threads that comprise much of the neurotransmitters and synapses through which messages are transported. Alcohol can cause this inner destruction and deposit harmful free radicals on these essential segments of your body. Alcohol can play havoc with your blood sugar levels. It can cause premature aging of body and mind. Avoid alcohol and you may very well avoid many of the debilities of so-called old age.

6. *Eat Several Small Meals During the Day.* This is preferable to three large ones to help give you an even level of blood sugar. It helps provide stabilized carbohydrate assimilation to give you day-long youthful energy and physical health.

7. *Eat a Protein Food on an Empty Stomach.* For breakfast, select a lean piece of meat, or fish, an egg, cheese, or seeds or nuts (chew them well). Just one or two portions is enough. *Benefit:* Hydrochloric acid secretion is increased after a night of fasting. In the morning, when your stomach is empty, the protein will be better metabolized and help control carbohydrate assimilation to give you day-long energy. Just a small piece of any of the above listed protein foods with a fresh fruit or vegetable salad, a whole grain bread product, and a caffeine-free bever-

age, will work wonders in keeping your blood sugar at an even level for the day ahead.

8. *Have Grains, Seeds, Nuts Daily.* Want a quick but long-lasting lift? Then munch on some whole grains or seeds or nuts. Just a handful is enough, or about a half cupful (approximately 3½ ounces). *Benefit:* These foods contain *pacifarins*, an antioxidant factor that builds your immunity to many ailments by strengthening your molecules and guarding against cross-linkage. They also contain *auxones*, substances that stimulate vitamin production. This protects against the onslaught of free radicals and begins an antioxidant reaction which guards against premature aging. *Suggestion:* In a plastic bag or box, keep an assortment of grains, seeds, and nuts available. Munch a tablespoon or two at a time. You will soon discover new feelings of youthful energy in body and mind, thanks to the antioxidant reactions of these foods.

9. *Enjoy More Raw Foods.* They are prime sources of valuable enzymes to help energize your entire being. Cooking changes protein into a form that could put free radicals in your system. Some nutrients, especially the B-complex and C vitamins are lost if food is cooked or boiled for a long amount of time. Raw foods call for more chewing; this releases additional enzymes that act to cleanse your molecules of oxidant particles and protect your cells against deterioration. *Suggestion:* Cook only those foods that, obviously, cannot be eaten raw. But eat all fruits, vegetables, whole grains, seeds, and nuts that can be eaten raw. This simple balance can work wonders in molecular rejuvenation.

10. *A Glass of Milk is Helpful.* Take a "milk break" when you are starting to feel the "jitters" or are going into that "slump." Milk is a rich source of protein and also contains a small amount of lactose, both of which will help maintain a stabilized blood sugar level. If you are not a milk fancier or are lactose-intolerant (unable to digest it), then opt for fermented milk such as buttermilk or yogurt. As an alternative, you could have a chunk or two of cheese with a whole grain cracker and a slice of fruit. You will be providing healthful protein and vitamins, as well as enzymes that keep antioxidant factors in check and your molecules at a good functional level.

11. *Honey Offers Moderate Rewards.* Honey should be raw, unrefined, unfiltered, and unheated. But remember, it is a sugar food, although it does have some nutrients (which are absent in sugar) and will help somewhat in maintaining a balanced blood sugar level. The rule here is moderation. That is, plan for one to two teaspoons of honey a day; one-half teaspoon at a time to sweeten herb tea or a caffeine-free

beverage or for any other use. But limit the intake of honey since in the process of metabolism, it, too, will create an acidifying reaction that could deposit oxidants and wastes that are harmful to your cells.

12. *Beat Fatigue with Buckwheat.* Its proteins are complete and of extremely high biological value in that they are comparable to proteins found in meat. Since buckwheat has *no* animal fat as in meat, it will give you a feeling of vigor, without the lethargy sometimes caused by eating meats. Have a bowl of buckwheat cereal or use buckwheat for baking, and you will soon discover how it can wipe away fatigue and make you feel youthfully energetic from head to toe.

13. *Awaken Energy with the Avocado.* This vegetable (botanically, it is a fruit) is a prime source of a seven-carbon sugar called *mannoheptulose* which helps suppress insulin production. While unwise for diabetics to eat, it is an excellent choice for those who have problems with hypoglycemia. The avocado will help pick up your fluctuating blood sugar level and keep it stable. At the same time, it contains vitamins that stimulate your body to help rid itself of the destructive free radicals. It may well be a miracle antioxidant food, and it's tasty, too. *Suggestion:* Use several slices of avocado on your raw vegetable salad daily. That's all. You will feel the difference almost at once.

14. *Take a Juice Break for Cellular Rejuvenation.* Fruits do contain concentrated forms of sugar that can cause speedy blood sugar upswings. This will happen with fruit juices, too—but only if consumed in great quantities. Therefore, plan to enjoy fresh fruits and their juices, but in moderation. *Good Choices:* banana, citrus fruits, strawberries, papaya, tart apples, fresh pineapple slices, fresh berries, grapefruit. *Choices to Use in Moderation:* These fruits have very high sugar levels and should be used sparingly. Included are grapes, dates, dried fruits (except if soaked in lots of water).

15. *Try Not to Mix Raw Fruits and Raw Vegetables at the Same Meal.* For some people, the different enzyme combinations in fruits and vegetables can be cellularly destructive. Poor digestion and gas are indications of the presence of oxidants and the outpouring of free radicals. If you experience this upset, it's best to keep these two desirable foods at a safe distance from each other. That is, eat fruits at one meal; then eat vegetables at a later meal. You may experience a healthy "lift" of vitality as your cells become free of congestion and your blood sugar levels become stabilized.

With the use of this simple 15-step program, you can help your body clock readjust internal timing devices so that a steady availability of blood sugar can give you a youthful feeling in body and mind.

## From "Always Tired" to "Speedball" in Three Days

David P. was becoming forgetful, not to mention irritable. As a computer operator he had many responsibilities but his edgy nerves, tremors, rapid heartbeat, and outbreaks of fatigue put his job in jeopardy. Although only in his early fifties, he looked and acted like a man twenty years older. He could not meet deadlines; he forgot appointments. At meetings he mumbled his words, dozed off at the conference table, was unable to put his thoughts in proper perspective. He might have been forced to retire, except that he consented to a checkup by an endocrinologist (glandular specialist).

His glucose tolerance test showed hypoglycemia. David P. was told to follow the preceding 15-step program. Anxious to restore his health and keep his job, he began the program at once. Within three days, his physical symptoms of fatigue and mental sluggishness vanished. He was now a "speedball" and worked with such youthful vitality he was put in for a promotion! Thanks to new-found molecular rejuvenation because of the 15-step program, David P. was rewarded with restoration of youthful energy.

# MIDDAY PICKUP

Because antioxidants are needed to combat the sluggishness caused by free radicals that cause the so-called "midday slump," you can erase such symptoms with a simple beverage that helps scour away these scavengers and rebuild your molecules within minutes.

In a glass of any citrus juice or combination of juices, stir in one spoonful of brewer's yeast and wheat germ. Blenderize for one minute. Drink . . .and within minutes, your slump will be gone and you will become a supercharged source of vitality.

*Benefits:* The vitamin C of the citrus juice boosts the antioxidant factors in brewer's yeast and wheat germ to scrub away free radicals from your cells so that you have speedy vitality. The "Midday Pickup" is refreshingly tasty, too.

# 60-SECOND EXERCISE BOOSTS ENERGY

Keep yourself in the pink. You need not undergo an exhausting gym workout (although it is helpful), but plan for a 60-second exercise right at home. This program helps oxygenate your system, wash away debris, and stabilize your blood sugar and blood pressure, too.

*Important:* Breathe normally. Plan on six seconds for each exercise. Count aloud to six and you'll keep track of the time and maintain normal breathing. Here's how:

1. Stand in a relaxed position, arms hanging loose. Don't clench your fists; don't bend your elbows or other joints.
2. Tense all your muscles at the same time as tightly as possible while breathing normally and counting aloud to six. You might try tensing each muscle group separately—legs, arms, chest, abdomen, face—and then try tensing them all at once. When you have done this, you should feel an immediate surge of vitality all over your body.
3. Relax and rest for a few seconds.
4. Repeat the exercise twice more.
5. Do this three times a day (morning, noon, and night).

Does four or five times a day sound like a lot? Remember, the entire set takes only 60 seconds . . .and that's little enough time to give you a powerhouse of healthy vitality.

## Erases Wrinkles, Glows with Youth, Sparkles with Joy within Two Days

Susan Q. worried when she saw the deep creases in her once youthful skin. She felt her energy slipping through her fingers, day after day. Life hardly had any joy. Each step was like a difficult mile. At times, her nerves were so edgy she would snap upon the slightest provocation. She had bouts of forgetfulness. At other times, her hands would start to tremble for no obvious reason. Susan Q. alienated her friends and family because of her erratic attitude. She felt she was aging very fast.

She agreed to be examined by a holistic or total body health practitioner, and took the glucose tolerance test. This confirmed suspicions about her sporadic behavior attitudes being due to uneven blood sugar levels.

Susan Q. consented to the 15-step program, but had to be closely supervised. Her health practitioner suggested someone make certain she followed the program carefully. In one day, she started to improve. By the end of the second day, her skin glowed with smoothness, and she had limitless energy, a firm grip, no more "shakes," and was a pleasure to be with. The 15-step program had cast out the grating free radicals, strengthened her molecules, nourished her neurotransmitter system so that she functioned with youthful smoothness and flexibility. She had been rescued from premature aging and was restored with a better memory and a desire to enjoy life.

## ANTIOXIDANT LUNCH FOR SUPER VIGOR AND HEALTH

To avoid afternoon slump or dull-witted lethargy, give your molecules a washing with antioxidant foods in the form of a tasty lunch. It's a great "pick-me-up" because these foods help protect against cross-linkage and damaging erosion through the presence of radicals.

**Easy, Effective, Energizing.** Just eat a 100 percent *raw* lunch. That's all! A good example would be a lunch containing such things as watercress, sprouts, seeds, and nuts. Or, have a chickpea spread (hummus, or mashed sesame seeds with chick peas) on whole grain bread. Add sprouts for a bigger boost in your blood sugar.

*Suggestion:* Have a platter of any desired and seasonal raw vegetables with, of course, sprouts for more effective molecular supercharging. That's all there is to it. This simple plan can have a dynamic reaction in putting new power into your network of neurotransmitters and molecular pathways and you can be filled with vitality and energy in minutes.

*Benefits:* The rich concentrations of enzymes and vitamins B-complex, C, and E, as well as an abundance of such minerals as calcium, copper, and magnesium in the raw foods set off a chain reaction within minutes. The free radicals are cast out of your system. Cell membranes are rebuilt. This helps improve muscular reflexes. Mental alertness is refreshed. The enzymes and nutrients of *raw* foods can give you a dynamic supercharging at midday . . . when you need it most. And it can last well into the evening, too!

Put a streak of youthfulness into your molecules by correcting your blood sugar level, ridding your body of the harmful free radicals, and nourishing your cells. You can enjoy immunity against aging with the 15-step program and antioxidant remedies and discover that life can be youthful again!

## HIGHLIGHTS

1. Enjoy improved energy by correcting any blood sugar imbalance with a corrective diet.

2. Avoid sugar, which is an oxidant, and can cause molecular clogging and a drop in energy levels. This simple step can work wonders in extending the prime of your life.
3. Have your blood sugar checked with a glucose tolerance test. It may well be the most important lifesaver you ever had!
4. Build the easy 15-step antioxidant program into your life to help rejuvenate your molecules and give you youthful, energetic health of body and mind.
5. David P. went from "always tired" to "speedball" in three days on this easy 15-step program. With rejuvenated molecules, he felt young again.
6. Wash away midday sluggishness with a tasty "Midday Pickup" tonic. It works in minutes to help you sparkle!
7. Try the 60-second exercise to revitalize your sluggishness.
8. Erase wrinkles and glow with sparkling youthfulness, as did Susan Q. when she followed the easy 15-step antioxidant program. It worked within two days.
9. Need a midafternoon pickup? Then enjoy it with the "Antioxidant Lunch!"

# 11

# Free Yourself from Salt–Sugar–Caffeine Addiction and Enjoy Total Rejuvenation

## Restores Youth by Eliminating Three Substances

Day after day, George S. felt his youthfulness slipping away from him in terms of lack of energy, sluggish reflexes, inability to concentrate on or participate in important activities. He had recurring nervous tremors; his blood pressure kept climbing. He had excessively high levels of blood fats. George S. could not control his weight gain and gave the appearance of being much older than he was. Someone called him "Gramps" behind his back when he was a long way from being worthy of that title!

His wife prevailed upon him to have a thorough checkup by a nutrition-minded physician. Reluctantly, he went through diagnostic tests. A new program emphasizing diet was prepared. He was told to make a few simple changes: eliminate all salt, sugar, and caffeine from his daily eating program. He had certainly overdone himself with these artificial stimulants and flavors, according to his diet chart.

Doubting that it would have an effect, George S. consented to please his wife and doctor. Within eight days, he felt more vitality. By the end of the twelfth day, his tremors ended; tests showed a normal blood pressure, weight, and blood fat level. His face became smooth; his eyes sparkled. He was such an image of youthful health by the end of the thirtieth day of this simple elimination diet, that a new co-worker asked why such a good-looking young man was not yet married! The fact is that this happily married man and father of three did look as young as his eldest teen-age son! The once-doubtful George S. became a firm believer in using nutritional correction to erase problems of so-

127

called aging. And it was all accomplished by eliminating the three cell-destroying evils: salt—sugar—caffeine!

You can help roll back the years, smooth out your skin, put the bloom of youthful roses back into your cheeks when you protect your body from age-causing free radicals that are brought on with the above-mentioned three substances. Let us take each one and see how they wreak destruction in your body and how to make simple changes to help you enjoy total rejuvenation.

## ARE YOU SALTING YOUR WAY TO PREMATURE OLD AGE?

*Problem:* Whether it comes from the shaker on your kitchen table or as an ingredient in packaged foods, salt can be a thief of life. It is believed to contribute to hypertension or high blood pressure. It puts an extra strain on the heart which can lead to cardiovascular problems, heart attack, stroke, or kidney failure. It may be involved in weight gain (salt absorbs water in your system), cause vertigo or dizziness and excessive thirst. It interferes with the transmission of nerve impulses and cellular health. One gram of sodium retains 50 grams of water in your body, and excessive water retention contributes to bloating and mineral imbalance. Over a period of time, it leads to tissue disintegration and the onset of aging. It can happen when you are in your twenties or thirties, or at any time of your life. Salt in any form can be a destroyer of your youth and lifespan.

**Hidden Sources of Salt.** It is found lurking in more places than the salt shaker. Most of the salt in foods is added to products during processing to help preserve and flavor them. It is added to vegetables in the canning and freezing process. It is used in smoking, curing, and processing of many meat products. Pickles and sauerkraut are preserved in brine (salt water) and are high in sodium. Most cheeses, mixes, sauces, soups, catsup, mustard, and salad dressings, as well as many breakfast cereals also have salt added.

Salt exists in not-so-obvious places, too. For example, baking powder and baking soda both contain salt, and are used in many cakes, cookies, and other baked goods. Salt is part of such ingredients as monosodium glutamate (MSG), sodium saccharin, sodium nitrate, sodium benzoate, sodium propionate, and sodium citrate. The word "sodium" as part of any ingredient listed in a label is your tip-off to the presence of this trouble-maker in your body.

**How Salt Can Cause Aging.** During digestion, salt becomes an acidic substance that erodes your molecular structures. Salt deposits the free radicals that become highly reactive and toxic chemical fragments that destroy healthy tissue. The salt-prompted substances then break down your primary genetic materials in your DNA–RNA cells and cause a form of cellular electrocution, so to speak. This is a form of internal disintegration that triggers off such symptoms of aging, faulty memory, weight gain, wrinkling of the skin, constant fatigue, and feelings of depression.

## EASY WAYS TO KICK THE SALT HABIT AND EXTEND YOUR PRIME OF LIFE

Begin today to cut back on salt in all forms. If you are a "salt addict," then you should follow some simple tricks that give you the tangy taste you desire, but eliminate the use of this troublesome substance. Try some of these easy ways to kick the salt habit:

1. Read labels and select products with lower or no salt content. Brands vary on the amounts of salt added to foods.
2. Start to eliminate the salt you add at the table a little bit at a time. Look for salt in recipes you prepare at home and cut it out. You do not need to salt the cooking water for vegetables, macaroni, rice, or other foods.
3. A drop of lemon juice can perk up the flavor of many foods. Try rubbing freshly cut ginger root on meat before barbequing. Fresh garlic adds zest to foods.
4. Bake your own cakes, cookies, and quick breads using sodium-free baking soda and powder, which is available in some pharmacies and health food or special diet food stores. Try making your own catsup, mayonnaise, and salad dressings without salt.
5. When possible, eat more fresh or plain frozen vegetables (without sauces), and eat vegetables canned without salt in place of regular canned vegetables.
6. Season foods with herbs, spices, lemon juice, and salt-free garlic and onion powders.
7. Taste food before you salt it. If you must add salt, try one shake instead of two.

8. At a restaurant, choose foods without sauces. If you prefer a sauce, ask for it "on the side" so you can control the amount. Ask to have your food served without added salt. Many dining places feature salt-free foods.
9. Peanut or olive oil provides a robust flavor to salad dressings and skillet dishes. It can take the place of salt.
10. Peppers and onions are so flavorful, they give dishes a no-salt-needed flavor. Try red bell peppers and onions such as shallots, chives, and leeks.
11. For a cracker spread with no salt, mix any of the following with softened unsalted butter or margarine: minced chives, grated lemon peel, ground red pepper, dill, your favorite herb or garlic powder. (No garlic salt, please!)

These are simple but effective tasty ways to help keep salt intake to a minimum. Remember, the less salt, the less free radicals, and the less aging!

### Lowers Blood Pressure, Overweight, Tension in Nine Days

The unusually high blood pressure reading, coupled with overweight and unrelieved nervous tension made Arlene O'B. worried about her health. Her dietician suggested that she eliminate salt in all forms. Switching to flavorful herbs and spices to satisfy her salt-addicted taste buds, Arlene O'B. was able to show lower readings, much lower weight, and a more relaxed temperament within nine days. Her molecular neurotransmitters became regenerated because they were free of the onslaught of the troublesome salt-caused free radicals. Arlene O'B. was given a new lease on life simply by saying "no" to salt in all its forms!

## SAY "NO" TO SUGAR AND "YES" TO A MORE YOUTHFUL LIFESPAN

*Problem:* Sugar is believed to be involved in problems of diabetes, tooth decay, heart disease, and related cardiovascular health problems. Sugar is also thought to be a cause of elevated levels of triglycerides or lipids (fatty substances) in the blood. These lesser-known fatty substances often take a back seat to cholesterol in terms of health risk, but sugar-created triglycerides do present problems in terms of raising fat levels in the bloodstream. Sugar interferes with the biological reactions of your molecules. They cause the formation of free radicals, the highly volatile broken-off molecular fragments that latch on to the other molecules and thereby bring on the signs of deterioration and aging. Sugar is also involved in excessive weight gain that can bring on a host of related problems. This mischief-making sweetener can be a threat to the length and health of your life.

**Hidden Sources of Sugar.** You would do well to dispose of the sugar bowl. So far, so good. But sugar is found in many processed and packaged foods. Labels may or may not list this sweetener. Sometimes, you may read "sugar added," other times, the presence of sugar is disguised in the list of ingredients such as: flavor, glucose, fructose, sucrose, maltose, corn syrup, "nutritive" sweeteners, caramel, to name a few. Much sugar comes from soft drinks. A typical 12-ounce can of soda contains about nine teaspoons of sugar.

If you purchase packaged products, they could also be sources of hidden sugar. For example, one slice of plain cake has six teaspoons of sugar; if iced, ten teaspoons. A one-and-a-half ounce candy bar has two teaspoons. One-half cup of sweetened cereal has about three teaspoons; one medium donut has three teaspoons and if glazed, six teaspoons. Fruit canned with syrup, just one-half cup gives you three teaspoons of sugar. One cup of ice cream has seven teaspoons. One slice of fruit pie has seven teaspoons. One cup of sherbet gives you fourteen teaspoons of sugar!

**How Sugar Causes Aging.** Bacteria in the body break sugar into acids which dissolve the protective covering of your molecules. As a prime example, this same acid dissolves the calcium from tooth enamel and paves the way to their decay. So it is with your molecular structures and your entire skeleton. Sugar causes erosion of the minerals that would otherwise help keep you youthfully healthy. Sticky sugar clings to your decaying bones and causes even further erosion. This gives rise to the fragmentary free radicals that cause destruction you can see in the form of aging. Your body's defense system breaks down. You become vulnerable to many illnesses and recovery is slower and slower. You could become "old" before your time because of the erosion caused by sugar.

# HOW TO SWEETEN YOUR LIFE
# WITHOUT THE USE OF SUGAR

Decide that your diet should be sweet, but in a natural form. You need not keep a gram-by-gram score of how much sugar is in the foods you eat. Instead, make some changes so that you consume less (or no) sugar from added sources. Some sweet tips are:

1. Use less of any sweetener, whether it be sugar, fructose, syrups, and so on. Gradually kick the habit.
2. When cooking, decrease the sugar in your favorite recipes by one-third to one-half.
3. At snack time, munch on fruits or fruit-sweetened yogurt (without sugar, please; read labels!).
4. For desserts, substitute fruit or milk desserts. Again, use no sugar.
5. If you do use canned fruits, select those that are canned in their own juices. If you still have the sweet habit, fruits canned in light syrup is favorable over heavy syrup.
6. Drink water instead of sweetened beverages during and between meals.
7. Try replacing soda pop with a mixture of half soda water and half fruit juice.
8. During a coffee break, at which you usually have a sugared beverage and a sweetened cake, make a change. Have a citrus fruit juice drink with a fresh apple instead of a pastry or donut. Your goal is to derive good health, not destructiveness, from your foods.
9. To nip the candy habit, have a portion of fruit or veggie chunks; or else, munch on salt-free seeds or nuts.
10. Instead of sweetened snacks, try to substitute fresh fruits and vegetables.

And remember, you can always use seasonings such as vanilla, cinnamon, carob, and concentrated berry juices as healthful replacements for the powdered white stuff we call "sweet sugar."

## Sugar Blues Cause Serious Woes for Body and Mind

"A bundle of nerves" was a good description of traffic manager Walter McF. He was always downing sweetened soda pop, munching on packaged cookies, frosted cupcakes, and other confections. His weight kept ballooning. He was so edgy, he would snap upon any provocation. His nerves were raw, most likely due to the destruction of calcium and other minerals in his body caused by sugar. Life was unbearable for himself and those around him.

A co-worker, who had gone through the same "sugarholic" condition, recognized the warning symptoms. A program of freedom from sugar was outlined for Walter McF. He began with some doubts; but in six days his weight began dropping and his moods became much sweeter. By the end of the second week he was cheerful again, could reason with others, and became a friend to his family and associates. By saying "no" to sugar, he kicked the habit. His molecular structure and neurotransmitter network healed. With the elimination of free radical overload, Walter McF. helped brighten up his body by casting out the sugar blues.

## CAFFEINE CAN BE A CUP OF CELLULAR COLLAPSE

*Problem:* Pharmacologists classify caffeine as a mild stimulant of the central nervous system and consider it to be one of the world's most widely used drugs. It can increase heartbeat and basal metabolic rate, promote secretion of stomach acid, and increase production of urine. It acts to dilate some blood vessels, and to constrict others. It has been implicated in such conditions as ulcers, heartburn, heart disease, cancer, fibrocystic breast disease, and birth defects. Caffeine stimulates the gastric mucosa and increases secretions of stomach acids, exacerbating existing ulcers. Caffeine consumption is also statistically linked with acute myocardial infarction (heart attack). There is also a link between bladder cancer and caffeine. So we see that caffeine from any source is a threat to your health.

**Hidden Sources of Caffeine.** The most commonly known source of caffeine comes from coffee. But this drug is also found in cocoa, milk chocolate, sweet chocolate, baking chocolate. It is in tea, many prescription and non-prescription medications for relief of pain and colds, and also in diet pills. A major source of caffeine is found in most soft drinks. Along with the sugar and salt (read labels), there is caffeine in soda pop, which makes it a triple threat to your health!

Decaffeinated beverages are not all that safe. The chemicals used to extract caffeine can be very destructive to your molecules. The most commonly used solvent is trichloroethylene which causes liver cancer in mice. Methylene chloride causes destruction of molecules and a spurt of free radicals that shoot throughout your body to create havoc and disintegration. There is concern that this solvent can predispose to cancer. With or without caffeine, certain beverages are undesirable, and other products containing caffeine are also full of risks.

**How Caffeine Causes Aging.** When it enters your system, caffeine upsets your metabolism. It causes your blood plasma to undergo undesirable changes. While in your bloodstream, the caffeine penetrates your body's tissues, extending throughout your entire system. In pregnant women, caffeine freely crosses the placenta and reaches the fetus, which may lead to birth defects. In men, caffeine enters the reproductive and prostatic fluids and can create molecular disintegration in these systems. By causing destruction of the molecular walls, there is an invasion of free radicals that can harm the DNA–RNA genetic materials. This can cause inner turmoil to the degree that it causes a breakdown of your basic functions. You can detect the ravages of the free radicals released by caffeine when you experience "coffee nerves"—anxiety, restlessness, poor sleep or frequent awakenings when asleep, headache, and heart palpitations. And these reactions can happen if you drink too many caffeine-containing sodas, cocoa, chocolate products, or tea beverages! You may not drink any coffee, but still have "coffee nerves" because of caffeine in the other products. Regardless of its source, caffeine is a drug that is destructive to your health. It can make you old before your time!

## HOW TO QUIT THE CAFFEINE ADDICTION AND ENJOY BETTER HEALTH

Be cautious of any coffee, tea or tea product, soda, or chocolate product. Even in small amounts caffeine can be destructive to your cells. Even the decaffeinated products have their risks because of the various solvents to remove the caffeine. These are harmful to your molecules and cause inner disintegration and aging. You have to quit being a caffeine addict by avoiding any of these products in any form. Besides, they all have sugar and salt or chemical substitutes that are undesirable for your basic health. Try some of these ways to break away from caffeine before it breaks your life:

1. Make your coffee or tea beverage weaker and weaker; that is, add more water and less of the product. This helps you ease out of the habit with fewer withdrawal symptoms.
2. Switch to fruit juices or fruit with milk. Or make a fruit fizz with club soda or seltzer water and fruit juice. Use it as a coffee substitute whenever the urge to drink something takes hold of you.
3. Spiced tomato juice or fruit juice punches (with no sugar) are good socializing drinks.
4. Discover the comforting warmth of herbal tea. Available in a variety of different flavors, herbal teas from your health food store or supermarket that are enhanced with a slice of lemon and a bit of honey, can make an excellent caffeine replacement as herbs are caffeine-free. Again, read labels.
5. Wake up in the morning to a cup of salt-free vegetable broth as a coffee replacement. Try a hot toddy: steamed apple juice with a sprinkle of cinnamon. These substitutes will energize you in moments and give you lasting vitality; in contrast, caffeine shocks your brain into alertness, gives you a dynamic explosion of energy, but then causes a letdown so you have a midday slump. Instead of coffee, you could have a fruit juice to provide healthful energy.

## Freedom from Caffeine = Freedom from Aging

A victim of overreacting to caffeine, Jennifer D.L. showed the ravages caused by this drug. Her skin had deep lines; she had telltale wrinkled bags under her eyes. She suffered from unrelieved anxiety, heart palpitations, and trembling hands. An embarrassing muscle twitch and uncontrollable spasms that made her wince constantly were upsetting to everyone. Close family members noted she was constantly drinking coffee and endless amounts of soft drinks. A neurologist was called in and he found she was a victim of not just "coffee nerves" but severe caffeine addiction. This drug had broken down her powers of resistance and immunity so that the outpouring of free radicals were destroying her millions of cells. These free radicals were attacking and disintegrating her barriers against illness. Jennifer D.L. was aging rapidly.

The neurologist gave her a simple prescription, so to speak. She was to take no caffeine or sugar or salt in any form! That was all. It was so simple, Jennifer D.L. doubted its effectiveness. Yet, she was desperate to regain her health and regain her fast-fading

youth, she followed this program. In eight days her skin
smoothed out; her muscular twitches subsided; spasms ended.
She was the picture of self-control. Her reflexes were stabilized;
she became alert again. She even started to look much, much
younger as the caffeine left her system and her molecular network
was regenerated. Now she could enjoy the best of life, free from
caffeine addiction!

## THE ANTIOXIDANT THAT HELPS YOU SLOW AGING AND SPEED HEALING

As you free yourself from the destructive elements of salt, sugar,
and caffeine, you will want to use antioxidants that are able to stave off
the effects of premature aging. They also help speed the knitting of the
cellular components and strengthen the molecular walls to resist the
impact of the free radicals. You can do this with the daily intake of one
most helpful antioxidant known as Vitamin E. It is the primary deter-
rent of free radical eruption in your body. You need this "booster shot"
of vitamin E when going off the salt, sugar, caffeine wagon.

**Sources of Antioxidant, Vitamin E.** In addition to a supplement which can be used in dosages approved by your health practitioner, you will find abundant amounts of vitamin E in wheat germ,
whole grains (brown rice, whole wheat oatmeal, cornmeal), asparagus,
sweet potatoes, beet greens, turnip greens, broccoli, and Brussels
sprouts. *Suggestion:* Plan to use as many of these foods as possible every
day in your meal program. You have been given a variety here to help
satisfy a finicky palate. So enjoy these foods as the antioxidant vitamin
E helps you enjoy a healthier body that is free of the effects of undesirable stimulants.

Live longer, live better, and most important, live younger with a
body and mind that are strengthened with the use of antioxidants.

## IN REVIEW

1. George S. experienced a restoration of youth by ending his use
   of salt, sugar, and caffeine.
2. Beware of salt because it can bring on premature old age.
3. Arlene O'B. was able to balance her blood pressure, lose
   weight, and melt tension in nine days by kicking the salt habit.

4. Sugar is a "sweet" way of getting old before your time. Get rid of this habit.
5. Walter McF. brightened up the sugar blues and corrected his body and mind disorders by eliminating sugar from his diet.
6. Caffeine can cause cellular collapse and should be avoided in all its forms.
7. Jennifer D.L. returned to the road to youth by giving up caffeine.
8. Boost the protective power of antioxidants with vitamin E products.

# 12

# How to Exercise Your Molecules and Feel Young All Over

Just 30 to 60 minutes a day of simple exercise will help revitalize the strength of your molecules and give your body the look and feel of total youth.

You can follow easy oxygenation or aerobic exercises in your own home, on the job, or during any brief amount of time. Within minutes, you will wash stale air from your body, keeping the free radicals from overpowering your molecules. Following easy fitness programs on a regular basis will help firm up your body and smooth out bulges. Most important, fitness will help rebuild and regenerate your molecules. You will be rewarded with inner immunity against the ravages of illness and so-called old age.

## AGING: ITS CAUSE AND EXERCISE: ITS ANTIOXIDANT

**Inactivity Is to Blame for Aging.** Inactivity or a sedentary way of life causes your molecules to become sluggish. Weakened, they become fragile and break apart. Fragments start to float all over your body. These fractions of molecules are the harmful and age-causing free radicals that have a single electron. The "glue" that holds all of your body molecules together consists of pairs of electrons. A free radical has only one electron and, therefore, is unstable. It causes damage to many of the biochemical structures of your body. But this is only the start of the aging process. Every time a free radical causes damage, it forms a new free radical. Therefore, the damaging effect continues on and on until aging sets in. This can happen when you are in your twenties or thirties if you allow yourself to become sedentary and disregard the importance of fitness.

**Exercise Is a Powerful Antioxidant.** You need to deactivate the process whereby free radicals reproduce. One powerful antidote is simple exercise or fitness. Yes, it can become an antioxidant. By flooding your body with important cleansing oxygen and accelerating your rate of respiration, deactivation (dismutation) of the toxic free radicals speeds up. Exercise will help slow down the formation and action of the free radicals; fitness will help wash these harmful substances out of your body and protect your molecules against disintegration and the onset of aging. This can happen within a few weeks of daily exercise programs done while sitting, standing, or walking, in almost any location where you have between 30 to 60 minutes of spare time. It's a small price to pay for a lifetime of youthfulness because of the antioxidant power of easy exercise.

**How Antioxidant Exercise Helps You Live Longer.** The antioxidant effect of exercise is to help your body grow new blood vessels so that your heart is thoroughly oxygenated and cleansed of the toxic free radicals. This helps overcome arteriosclerosis by scrubbing free radicals out of your clogged arteries. At the same time, the antioxidant power of exercise helps your blood vessels grow in size, thus enabling blood to flow more smoothly through them. This reaction will help lower your blood pressure and protect against heart problems. If you exercise daily, causing your arteries to expand, there is less risk that a clot will obstruct blood flow. In effect, regular fitness can help make you immune to cardiovascular disorders so that you live not just longer, *but younger!* Ready?

## BEFORE YOU BEGIN

If you are over age 30, a visit to your family physician is suggested prior to beginning your program. This is especially important if you have been inactive for a period of time, are more than 10 pounds overweight, or have any medical problem.

**Warm Up First.** Prepare your muscles for the activity to follow. A warm-up helps boost your respiration and prepare your molecular system for the antioxidant reaction of the fitness program. Simple stretching helps ease stress and tension in your muscles, making them more pliable.

**Five to Ten Minutes.** Give your body a chance to limber up within this time slot so antioxidants work more effectively in deactivating the free radicals. Start at a medium pace and gradually increase by the end of the 5–10 minute warm-up period. Below are three easy warm up exercises. Each one helps stretch different parts of your body. Remember, do these stretching exercises slowly and in a steady, rhythmical way. You'll be preparing your body for the rejuvenating effect of the alerted antioxidants.

1. *Wall Push:* Stand about 1½ feet away from the wall. Then lean forward, pushing against the wall, keeping your heels flat. Count to 10, then rest. Repeat one or two times.

2. *Palm Touch:* Stand with your knees slightly bent. Then bend from your waist and try to touch your palms to the floor. Do not bounce. Count to 10, then rest. Repeat one to two times. *Note:* If you have low back problems, do this warm-up with your legs crossed.

3. *Toe Touch:* Place your right leg level on a stair, chair, or other slightly raised object. Keeping your other leg straight, lean forward and slowly try to touch your right toe—with the right hand 10 times and with the left hand, 10 times. Do not bounce. Now switch legs and repeat with each hand. Repeat entire exercise one or two times.

*Suggestions:* During the warm-up, perform each stretch slowly, smoothly, and comfortably. Do *not* bounce because this can tear or strain your muscles and give rise to more free radical problems because of fragmented tissues. Breathe deeply while you perform each movement and as you hold each stretch. Never stretch to the point of feeling pain. Alternative warm-ups could include rhythmic activities, jogging in place, arm circles, or hip rotations.

*Benefits:* The warm-ups oxygenate your respiratory and cardiovascular systems to send forth an antioxidant reaction that helps your arteries become more elastic, balance your cholesterol levels, more efficiently eliminates lactic acid (a substance that can cause fatigue and tension) from your muscles, and improves your blood health.

## CHECK ANTIOXIDANT POWER THROUGH YOUR TARGET ZONE

Are the antioxidants washing away free radicals? Are they helping to restore the youthful strength of your molecules. You can find out by keeping track of your target zone, or your heart rate. Your maximum heart rate is the fastest your heart can beat. Exercise above 75 percent of the maximum heart rate may be too strenuous. Exercise below 60 percent gives your heart and lungs little conditioning and weak antioxidant benefit.

The best antioxidant activity level is 60 to 75 percent of this maximum rate, which is called your *antioxidant target zone.*

*When You Begin:* Aim for the lower part of your zone (60 percent) during the first few months. As you get into better shape, gradually build up to the higher part of your zone (75 percent). After six months or more of regular exercise, you can work out at up to 85 percent of your maximum heart rate, if you wish.

**Your Personal Rate.** Monitor your activity by keeping your heart rate within a "training rate" range. To find your target zone, look for the age category closest to your age and read the line across. *Example:* If you are 30, your target zone is 114 to 142 beats per minute. If you are 43, the closest age on the chart is 45; the target zone is 105 to 131 beats per minute.

*Note:* Your maximum heart rate is usually 220 minus your age. The preceding figures are average and should be used as general guidelines.

*Careful:* A few high blood pressure medicines lower the maximum heart rate and thus the target zone rate. If you are taking hypertension medications, ask your physician if your fitness program needs to be adjusted for your personal needs.

*At a Glance:* To deduce your personal antioxidant target zone,

| Age | Target Zone (60–75%) | Average Maximum Heart Rate–100% |
|---|---|---|
| 20 years | 120–150 beats per minute | 200 |
| 25 years | 117–146 beats per minute | 195 |
| 30 years | 114–142 beats per minute | 190 |
| 35 years | 111–138 beats per minute | 185 |
| 40 years | 108–135 beats per minute | 180 |
| 45 years | 105–131 beats per minute | 175 |
| 50 years | 102–127 beats per minute | 170 |
| 55 years | 99–123 beats per minute | 165 |
| 60 years | 96–120 beats per minute | 160 |
| 65 years | 93-116 beats per minute | 155 |
| 70 years | 90–113 beats per minute | 150 |

subtract your age from 220 and take 70 to 85 percent of the resulting figure. *Examples:* A 20-year old man has a maximum heart rate of 200. His target zone would be 140 (70 percent) to 170 (85 percent) beats per minute heart rate. However, a 65-year old man with a maximum attainable heart rate of 150 beats per minute would have a target zone of 107 (70 percent) to 130 (85 percent) beats per minute.

## HOW TO COUNT YOUR PULSE

Your pulse count is nearly always the same as the number of heart beats per minute (the heart rate). When you stop exercising, quickly place the tips of two or three fingers on one hand just below the base of your thumb on the inside of your wrist of your other hand. Apply light pressure to feel the beat. (Do *not* use your thumb since it has a pulse of its own that can be confusing.) Count your pulse for 30 seconds and multiply by two.

If your pulse is below your target zone, exercise a little more vigorously the next time. If you're above your target zone, exercise a little easier. If it falls within your target zone, you're doing fine. The antioxidants are at full force in rebuilding your molecular structure.

*Important:* Count your pulse immediately upon stopping the particular exercise because the rate changes very swiftly once exercise is either slowed or stopped.

Once you're exercising within your target zone, check your pulse at least once each week during the first three months and periodically thereafter. If you have any problems, such as difficulty in breathing, or you experience faintness or prolonged weakness during or after an exercise, you are doing it too hard. Simply cut back and check your pulse to see if you are still within your target zone. Looking ahead, as the antioxidants restructure your molecules and you start to look and feel much younger, increase the vigor of the exercise so as to benefit from intensified antioxidant reaction. But be sure to keep your heart rate in the target zone for at least 20 minutes so that this cell-molecular rebuilding program can be established.

## SETTING UP YOUR SCHEDULE

Your goal should be a minimum of 30 to 60 minutes every single day. You may start out with the 30-minute goal and gradually increase it to 60 minutes. Your activity should be brisk, sustained, and regular.

Do not push yourself to the point where it is no longer any fun, but stick to it, if you can.

If you've eaten a meal, hold off exercising for at least two hours so that the antioxidants can work without interfering with the digestive process. Otherwise, do your antioxidant exercise program first, and eat one hour afterwards.

## COOL-DOWN LAST FOR TOP-NOTCH ANTIOXIDANT EFFECT

After your exercise program, allow your body to experience a gradual cool-down so that the antioxidant effect of cleansing out the free radicals and strengthening your immunity reserves will be able to reach its full potential. Be careful not to come to an abrupt stop because this can cause free radical backup. This is a clogging together of free radicals to create congestion. Instead, give your heart, lungs, and muscles a chance to adjust. To cool down, try some mild stretching, deep breathing, and walking as you swing your arms.

You can also cool down by changing to a less vigorous exercise such as from jumping rope to walking. Swim more slowly towards the end of your exercise session. If you have been running, end by walking briskly. Just try to stretch and relax your muscles so the antioxidants can work without the impediment of congestion. Basically, a cool-down period of just 10 to 15 minutes after your exercise will assist in slowly returning your body back to normal function. A cool-down helps your antioxidants transport blood from your exercised muscles back to your heart and protects you against muscle and joint soreness.

To help release antioxidants within your system that will restore strength and integrity to your molecular fortress of youthfulness, here is a set of easy, but effective, fitness programs you can do just about anywhere. Mix and match them to suit your tastes, but aim for a minimum of 30 to 60 minutes each day. You will know they are producing their cell-building reconstruction when you test your pulse to see whether you are within your personal target zone (shown on the table on page 141). You will see the results in a livelier step, a youthful appearance, and a glow of total health.

**Neck Exercise.** Sit in a chair, arms and shoulders relaxed. Start with head to one side. Slowly drop head forward and move it across your chest in a smooth semicircle until facing the other side.

Repeat. Movements should be gentle and controlled to avoid strain or dizziness.

**Shoulder Release.** Sit or stand tall, arms relaxed. Shrug shoulders up toward ears and relax them down. Rotate your shoulder in one direction s-l-o-w-l-y, making two or three complete rotations. Rotate shoulders the other direction up to five times.

**Hamstring Stretch.** Sit with one knee bent and the other leg resting on a chair or table of the same height. Keeping your leg straight, gently bend forward from your waist until a comfortable stretch is felt. Hold. Repeat with your other leg.

**Hip Stretch.** Sit on one side edge of a chair. Exhale as you bring your outside knee toward your chest. Return foot to floor and inhale as you extend your leg back as far as possible. Alternate legs.

**Trunk Twist with Arm Stretch.** Stretch one arm to your side with palm facing back. Slowly twist head, shoulder, arm, and trunk to side and back as far as is comfortable for you. Hold for five seconds, then relax. Repeat on other side.

**Roll Down.** Sit with knees bent, hands resting on knees, and chin tucked in to chest. Exhale as you s-l-o-w-l-y lower your body down: first back, then shoulders, then head, to touch floor. Knees remain bent throughout. Use your arms to assist returning to sitting position. Repeat.

**The Curl Up.** Lie on your back, knees bent, feet flat on the floor, arms relaxed at sides. Press the small of your back flat to the floor. Lift your head and shoulders off the floor and look toward your knees while exhaling. Relax and repeat. *Tip:* When you have sufficient strength, curl up to a sitting position, exhaling as you do.

**Single Knee Tuck.** Lie on your back, one leg straight and one leg bent. Keeping bent leg still, grasp hands behind your other knee and pull it toward your chest while exhaling. Hold. Return to sitting position. Alternate legs and repeat. Your lower back and head should remain on the floor throughout.

**Side Leg Raises.** Lie on one side with your head resting comfortably on your extended arm, your other arm and hand resting on the floor in front of your waist (to maintain balance). Your bottom leg should be bent at your knee to protect your back. Exhale as you slowly raise your top leg; inhale as you slowly lower it. Your top leg should remain straight and your toes should point forward throughout. Repeat on your other side.

### Thirty Minutes a Day Brings Freedom from Arthritis Stiffness

For years, Joel E. B. was troubled with such arthritic stiffness, he could scarcely hold a spoon without pain. Bending to tie his shoelaces brought spasms of pain that made him cry out as he tried to straighten up. He had gone the route of chemotherapeutic injections which gave him side effects that were worse than his disorder. He was just told to live with his arthritic-like disability.

A health magazine featuring an article on how exercise can boost antioxidant vigor to correct metabolic disorders such as his condition, alerted Joel E. B. to this possible means of help.

He located a physical therapist who explained that much inflammatory pain, soreness, and swelling could be traced to injury of the ligaments connected to the muscles. This triggered an inflammatory response that automatically produced free radicals. These trouble-makers delayed and halted healing of the injured ligaments and the inflammatory process continued to cause arthritic-like stiffness. The treatment? To boost antioxidants via exercise to cast out the free radicals and permit healing to continue.

Joel E. B. was told about the 30-minute minimum exercise schedule; he also found out about reaching the antioxidant target zone. He followed an assortment of the preceding exercises. Within eleven days, his inflammatory swelling and pain went down. His limbs became more flexible. His hands were so firm and strong, he could work at his machine shop hobby again. He could bend and twist in all directions with nary a spasm. By the end of the twentieth day, he said goodbye to painful injections and risky drugs; he also bid his arthritic-like pain goodbye. The antioxidants had helped him recover!

# SIMPLE DAY-TO-DAY ANTIOXIDANT FITNESS METHODS

You may say you do not have time for exercise. But if you keep yourself active, you will help boost antioxidant levels so that you can build an inner fortress against the ravages of age-causing free radicals.

Here is a set of no-fuss, effective fitness methods that will help keep your degree of immunity at a high level.

1. Walk . . . walk . . . walk! Park your car a few blocks from your destination and walk the rest of the way. If possible, plan to take a 30- or 60-minute walk after each of your major meals.
2. Use your feet instead of the elevator. Take to the stairwells, slowly, but regularly. You will help strengthen your cardiovascular and respiratory systems.
3. Keep moving when you talk on the phone. Stand up. Move and walk around as far as the phone cord permits.
4. Try a stomach press: Clasp your hands together and place your palms against your slightly pulled-in stomach. Tense up your stomach muscles. Press your hands firmly against the tightened stomach muscles. Count to ten and relax. Repeat frequently.
5. Try moving walls: Stand one pace away from the wall. Place your hands against the wall at shoulder height. Press forcefully as if you could move the wall. Count to ten and relax. Do this often to create rhythmic exercise while standing in one position.
6. Switch on a record or tape with frantic dance music. For 10 or 15 minutes, exercise to the wild breakdance or go-go style or whatever is current. Rock and roll, twist and turn, reach and stretch. The more imaginative, the more effective. Give your entire body a workout. Let the music keep you go-go-going without interruption. It's a fun way to exercise and help boost antioxidant effectiveness.
7. Before you go out the door in the morning, straighten up. Stand tall, clasp hands behind neck. Pull elbows up and back and hold. Do it three times, luxuriating in the pull.
8. Spread feet wide apart. Extend arms forward, elbows straight. Raise your arms up, brushing your ears with your shoulders. Bring your arms down behind you in a circle. Try five times and work up to ten.
9. Shake yourself loose and try one more: Stand correctly, shoulders and hips pressed against the wall; feet about six inches from the wall. Drop your upper body limply forward, bending at your hips. Relax. Return to starting position. Once more. And again.
10. Try rope skipping, it's a great way to flood your system with refreshing antioxidants. All you need is a jump rope, or any six-foot length of rope. Try jumping with two feet, then alternate right and left feet on each turn of the rope for five minutes, stopping when winded.

11. Do you sit behind a desk all day? While doing so, raise your right buttock and hold for a count of five. Lower. Raise the left buttock and repeat.
12. Drop a pencil to the floor at your left side. With your back straight, slide left hand down your body and retrieve it. Next, drop the pencil to your right, sliding your right arm down to pick it up. Repeat five times.
13. As you read anything (at home or at work), push you chair back from your desk. Slip the toes of one foot through the handle of a purse or briefcase and, holding your leg straight, lift. Repeat ten times without touching the floor; then switch to the other foot. *Alternative:* Grasp a wastebasket between your ankles and lift, squeezing ankles together at the same time.

# HOW TO TRANSFORM HOUSEWORK INTO ANTIOXIDANT EXERCISE

1. Dust in the high places, on tiptoes, stretching. Lift your rib cage, tuck in your tummy, pinch in your derrière.
2. Dust in low places, squatting instead of bending. Hold on to the table leg if you must, but keep your back straight as you bend from your hips.
3. When washing floors on all fours, keep your back parallel to the floor. Slide forward, head down, as you scrub in sweeping arcs.
4. With feet apart, grasp dustcloth between both hands over your head. Pull the cloth from side to side, bending in the direction of the pull. Keep your back straight.
5. Hold dustcloth at shoulder height. Inhale. Raise arms straight and bend forward from your waist. Exhale.
6. After polishing each dining room chair, rest your hands on the back, bend down from your knees, then rise up on your toes.
7. Grip the same chair with your left hand, left leg on the floor. Lift your right leg to your side and swing forward and back. Make circles. Turn around and repeat with your left leg.

Exercising while you do housework may sound like a double dose of punishment, but you do have to clean. If you combine it with exercise, the antioxidant reaction will make you feel twice as good afterwards. And . . . you thought housework was for the birds!

## Firms Up Flab, Loosens Limbs, Erases Stiffness

Edna DeF. had a part-time job and was a most-of-the-time housekeeper. She had little time for fitness. When she began to show unsightly bulges and began to have stiff limbs, she enrolled in a small fitness group. She not only did exercises at the health club, but also at work, while waiting for a commuter bus, while sitting, and (especially) while doing housework. She followed many of the preceding programs. In just seven days, her flab became firm and she had youthful flexibility of her arms and legs. The antioxidants created by fitness had cast out the harmful free radicals. Edna DeF. jokes that she looks forward to housework because it keeps her looking so young. And it does!

With the use of easy exercises, you, too, can deactivate harmful and age-causing free radicals. Just 30 to 60 minutes a day can add up to many more decades of youthful health.

# IN REVIEW

1. Boost your powers of immunity against aging with the use of antioxidants released through simple daily exercise and fitness programs.
2. Follow the guidelines given in the chapter on the warm-up, how to check your antioxidant target zone, and the cool-down.
3. Plan for 30 to 60 minutes daily of the assorted easy fitness programs to help you look and feel younger. As antioxidants improve your body, you will feel more energetic, stronger, younger, and better overall. You will appreciate the rewards of regular fitness.
4. Joel E.B. was rescued from addiction to medicines because of arthritic-like stiffness and pain by using fitness to boost antioxidant healing reactions.
5. Edna DeF. used a variety of fitness tips when standing, sitting, at work, or doing housework. Within weeks, she was free of her flab, had flexible limbs, and looked great, too, thanks to antioxidants.

# 13

# How to Wake Up Your Glands for Total Youth

You are as young and healthy as your glands. When these youth builders release energy-producing hormones that act as antioxidants to rebuild your cells and organs, you will be filled with the joy of daily living. With proper stimulation, you can wake up your glands to release these essential hormones to help your body and mind glow with the springtime of youthful health.

To understand how to use simple nutritional programs to boost the release of sufficient antioxidants, here is a brief explanation of these dynamic sources of rejuvenation from within.

## YOUR GLANDULAR SYSTEM

A gland is an organ which manufactures a substance to be utilized elsewhere in your body. If this secretion goes directly into your bloodstream, the gland is part of your endocrine system. If this secretion goes through a duct or tube to surrounding tissues, the gland is part of your exocrine system, such as your sweat glands. Your set of endocrine glands include the adrenals, pituitary, thyroid, pancreas, and sex glands. These are your most valuable antioxidant-producing organs.

## YOUR HORMONE SYSTEM

The antioxidant secretions released by glands are called *hormones*. They are like "fountains of youth" in that they influence your growth, development, and even your behavior to some extent. Some glands reg-

149

ulate body chemistry, while still others control the contraction of muscle tissues. There are antioxidant hormones that influence various sex functions. Still others will help cast out free radicals to help you control weight levels, guard against allergies, arthritis, diabetes, errors in metabolism, and give you a youthful skin.

**Each Hormone Has a Specific Function.** When your gland releases a hormone, it is directed to perform a very specific and singular function. It cannot do the job of another hormone. When it has accomplished its objective, it is prepared for elimination. When the specific hormone is needed again, the glands will be called upon to make it available. So you see that you need healthy glands to have antioxidant hormones available upon demand. Small wonder that glands are considered the "masters" of youthful health.

## CAUTION: FREE RADICALS CAN CLOG GLANDS AND BLOCK FULL HORMONE RELEASE

During the metabolic process of digestion, molecular fragments break off to form the noxious free radicals. Many of these errant pieces cling to your glands to create blockages that can reduce the release of important antioxidant hormones. Some causes of these accumulations of wastes are consumption of highly refined foods such as bleached flour products, hard animal fats, sugar, salt, chemical preservatives, and additives. Other sources of free radical buildup come from the sediment in the air you breathe, the fallout in the water you drink. Your glands are under a constant assault from these pollutants.

*Problem:* A waste-clogged gland will be so choked up, it comes to a virtual halt. A trickle of hormone serves to keep you barely functioning. Denied an adequate supply of antioxidant hormones, your body ages. You have symptoms such as aging skin, allergies, diabetes or blood sugar upset, and loss of immunity to illness. You can age well before your time if your glands are overpowered by free radicals and waste molecules and the supply of hormones are cut off.

**For Total Youth: Total Glandular Cleansing.** If the vitality of just one gland is impaired, the antioxidant activity of that plus other glands (as well as organs and tissues) become seriously affected.

Your goal is to achieve total youth through total glandular cleansing. You can do this with everyday foods that help scrub away the free radicals and put "go power" into your glands. You can wash out and wake up your endocrine system so your entire body responds with joyful health.

## CLEAN ADRENALS = FREEDOM FROM ALLERGIES, ARTHRITIS, STRESS

Shaped like Brazil nuts, the adrenals are a pair of glands which sit astride each kidney. The adrenals release such antioxidant hormones as epinephrine and norepinephrine which help cast out free radicals and stimulate your heart, balance your blood pressure, regulate hypoglycemia to control blood sugar reactions, and stabilize your stress levels to help you cope with emergency or tension-filled reactions. These same steroid-like antioxidant hormones protect against joint-muscle-artery sedimentation which might otherwise cause arthritic symptoms. A healthy pair of adrenals will release androgen hormones to cause large masses of muscle tissue to promote healthy strength.

**Controls Aging.** The adrenal antioxidant hormones boost blood levels of *cortisol.* This is a valuable substance that guards against the accumulation of a free radical cluster known as *melanin-stimuli hormones* (MSH). Cortisol controls overproduction so that the MSH waste does not overpower cells and tissues to cause aging.

**Keeping Your Adrenals Clean.** The delicate tubules and channels of your adrenals need to be cleansed of free radicals so they are able to release sufficient amounts of antioxidant hormones to maintain youthful health. *Examples:* You need pantothenic acid (a component of B-complex) to help strengthen the cortex segment (covering) against the invasion of the free radicals. You also need vitamin C to protect against cellular breakdown and to nourish the minuscule tissues so they resist invading fragments. A combination of *both* of these nutrients will cleanse your adrenals and energize this pair of glands to release important immunity-building hormones.

**Adrenal Cleanser Tonic.** In a glass of fresh citrus juice, add one teaspoon of brewer's yeast (from supermarket or health food store), and a half teaspoon of honey, if desired. Stir or blenderize. Drink one glass at noontime. Drink another freshly prepared glass in late-afternoon.

*Antioxidant Benefits:* The rich concentration of pantothenic acid and vitamin C join together to scrub and regenerate your adrenal cells and tissues. The honey speeds up the action. Within moments, an invigorated and cleansed adrenal will release powerful adrenalin and cortisol, as well as the valuable stress-protecting epinephrine and norepinephrine. You will experience more agility in your arms and legs, you will have greater resistance against allergies, you will be immune to much stress, thanks to the release of antioxidants to deactivate free radicals. Just two glasses daily of the refreshing "Adrenal Cleanser Tonic" will wake up your adrenals to help give you super health.

## Reverses Aging, Ends Arthritis, Soothes Nervousness

As a landscape designer, Howard A. J. was understandably worried when he found it difficult to move his arms and legs. Straightening up after some bending gave him an arthritic pain in his lower back. He tired quickly. He was sensitive, jumping at any noise or activity, however mild. He walked with a stiff gait. His creeping "old age" threatened his means of livelihood. And Howard A. J. was not even in his fifties. Noticing his stooped movements, an endocrinologist client of Howard's suggested he wake up his sluggish adrenals. He recommended more B-complex and C vitamins. But for immediate adrenal-cleansing and antioxidant-boosting action, Howard A. J. was told to drink two glasses daily of the "Adrenal Cleanser Tonic." Within three days, the supercharging of antioxidant hormones via clean adrenals made a welcome difference. He looked more alert. He had full flexibility of his arms and legs and developed good posture, too. He could bend like a youthful acrobat. He was calm and responsive. He had youthful energy. The "Adrenal Cleanser Tonic" had lived up to its name. He felt reborn!

**Adrenal-Nourishing Foods.** These are valuable brewer's yeast, all citrus fruits and their juices, whole grains in cereals and breads, fresh fruits and vegetables as well as their juices. These are powerhouses of adrenal-invigorating nutrients that will boost an abundant supply of hormones. You can actually eat and drink and grow younger with these foods.

## CLEAN PITUITARY = WEIGHT CONTROL, CIRCULATION, ENERGY

Situated at the base of your brain, this pea-sized gland is linked by a stalk to your thinking organ. Often called the "master gland," a clean pituitary controls almost all body functions via a network of hormones. These hormones control your weight, blood circulation, and energy capacity. Situated in your pituitary is your *hypothalamus,* or appetite control center. If cleansed of free radicals, this part of your pituitary protects you against the urge to overeat. A clean pituitary is able to release *somatotropin* (body growth hormone); *corticotropin* (adrenal stimulating hormone); *FSH, LSH* and *prolatin* (which stimulate the ovaries, uterus, and breasts respectively in women); vasopressin (controls retention of water in the body and protects against mineral loss by promoting their reabsorption in the kidneys). These functions influence your health from head to toe, hence the "master gland" designation.

**Keeping Your Pituitary Clean.** Lots of fresh water and juices (sugar-free and salt-free, please) help wash away free radicals that might otherwise impinge upon the pituitary's ability to release valuable hormones.

**Magnesium Scrubs Your Pituitary.** Found in nonprocessed nuts, whole grain foods, dark green vegetables, and soy products, this mineral is a powerful pituitary-scrubber. It acts as an intracellular electrolyte which combines with *ATP* (adenosine triphosphate), a substance that has antioxidant cleansing power. Magnesium plus ATP will wash free radicals out of the cellular chambers of your pituitary; this creates an electrolyte energizing effect, causing this master gland to release a shower of youth-building hormones.

**Pituitary Power Salad.** On a plate of fresh green leafy vegetables, add cooked dried beans, chopped nuts, a sprinkle of wheat germ. Try diced celery, too. A bit of apple cider vinegar and lemon juice provide the tangy taste. Plan to eat this "Pituitary Power Salad" each day. Vary the cooked dried beans and nuts and vegetables to have a new treat each day. Before long, this high-magnesium salad will regenerate your pituitary to release antioxidant hormones that will make you look and feel young all over.

### Loses Weight, Boosts Circulation, Feels Revitalized

Feeling mentally and physically tired, seeing her hips and thighs spreading, Doris D'A. felt understandably depressed. Ordinary housework was a chore. Meals were tardy or improperly prepared. Everyone whispered how Doris D'A. was sliding downhill. A neighbor suggested that she see a local gland specialist as she suspected this could be the source of her problem. A checkup showed an underactive pituitary gland. It needed to be cleansed of free radicals so its regulating hormones could gush forth to provide health-boosting benefits. Doris D'A. was told to take magnesium supplements daily, to use magnesium-rich foods, and to eat the potent and tasty "Pituitary Power Salad." Within two days, she felt her weight dissolving. Her circulation improved; energy was restored. Eight days later, after the magnesium supplement and salad program, she had an enviable trim figure again, and was a bundle of energy. When someone said she was back to her "old self," she corrected them to say she was now her "young self " once more!

**Magnesium Is a Powerful Pituitary Energizer.** Magnesium from a supplement or foods is a dynamic energizer of the pituitary gland. Magnesium is an electrolyte, that is, its molecules carry a small electrical charge called a magnesium ion. This substance stimulates the contraction and relaxation of your pituitary, thus deactivating the accumulated free radicals. This same magnesium ion uses its antioxidant power to revitalize your pituitary. This supplies the required hormones needed for weight control, healthy circulation, and overall good feeling.

# CLEAN THYROID = YOUTHFUL METABOLISM, STRONG CELLS, LONGER LIFE

Butterfly-shaped, this is a two-part gland that rests against the front of your windpipe. The thyroid gland releases *thyroxin,* a valuable hormone that uses its antioxidant power to regulate the metabolism of your billions of body cells. This hormone stabilizes the rate of glucose absorption (which influences energy) and also cellular nourishment. It is involved in maintaining a balanced body temperature. If your thyroid becomes clogged with free radicals, it releases too much thyroxin in a frantic effort to overcome the sedimentation, then you may lose too much weight, show a rapid pulse and breathing rate, or suffer from extreme nervousness. Or, if the thyroid is too polluted with the free radicals, it may release too little thyroxin; this inhibits growth, causes dry or aging skin, and a slowdown of body-mind reaction. So you need a clean thyroid, free of molecular wastes in order to provide a steady and balanced supply of youth-restoring antioxidant hormones.

**Keeping Your Thyroid Clean.** The valuable mineral, iodine, is dynamic in its ability to cause antioxidant reactions that shake loose and wash out accumulated free radicals. Your thyroid uses iodine to manufacture the hormone, thyroxine, which is a powerful antioxidant that pours into your bloodstream to rejuvenate your cells, regulate your metabolism, and help protect against overload of cellular pollutants. Your thyroid may well be the "gate keeper" of your body's health.

## WHY OCEAN-BORNE FOODS
## ARE SUPER THYROID CLEANSERS

From the briny depths of the oceans, certain edibles contain iodine that is needed to keep your thyroid in good shape. Seafood, of course, is a prime source of this miracle mineral. Also, sea salt or kelp (available at health food stores), along with seaweed as a vegetable, will provide your thyroid with this important mineral. You can actually eat your way to a healthier thyroid with the iodine in seafood and seaweed products.

Plan to have freshly prepared seafood at least twice weekly. It provides you with rich concentrations of iodine to alert your thyroid to produce its cleansing antioxidant reaction via the thyroxine hormone. Within minutes after eating these foods, a total cellular regeneration takes place. You will look and feel refreshingly young within a short while.

**Thyroid Tonic.** To a glass of tomato juice, add just one-quarter teaspoon of kelp. Add a squeeze of lemon juice for a better flavor, if desired. Stir vigorously. Drink just one such "Thyroid Tonic" each day. You will feel the joy of life as free radicals are cleansed and your thyroid can function freely.

## Balances Weight, Becomes Calm, Overcomes Laziness

Gerald LaM. had a "yo-yo" battle with his weight. It came on; it went off; it came back on again. He fell victim to bouts of nervous anxiety. He could hardly control his outbursts of temper. Then he would become slow-moving, even lazy. His stockroom supervisor job was being jeopardized. He felt fit to be tied. At times, others wanted to do just that to keep him under control.

A company nutritionist diagnosed his condition as a free radical-clustered thyroid. Sporadic production of thyroxin (a valuable antioxidant hormone) was responsible for his seesaw behavior and up-and-down weight levels. George LaM. was told to take the "Thyroid Tonic" daily to provide cleansing of the gland and iodine nourishment. Within three days he began to slim down and keep weight off. By the fourth day he began to feel restored energy. At the end of six days he was a changed person. He had a slim-trim shape, a pleasant disposition and a feeling of total rebirth. Thanks to the antioxidant action of his newly cleansed thyroid, his iodine-invigorated thyroxin hormone could keep him in tip-top health.

**A Clean Thyroid Is Up to You.** Schedule seafoods and kelp as part of your menu plan. You will be boosting your iodine intake and keeping your thyroid clean of free radicals. A regular supply of thyroxin also helps protect you against lassitude, mental dullness, weight irregularities, and general malaise. A sprinkling of kelp tonight . . . and a youthful thyroid-nourished body is yours tomorrow morning!

## CLEAN PANCREAS = HEALTHY SUGAR METABOLISM, IMPROVED DIGESTION

A large, long organ or gland (called sweetbread in animals), it is located behind the lower part of your stomach. Your pancreas performs two vital functions. (1) It regulates glucose production, whereby it releases insulin needed to take glucose into cells, synthesize glycogen in the liver, and distribute glycogen to all body parts. (2) It releases insulin from the isles of Langerhans, small cells within the pancreas. *Important:* A pancreas free of harmful fragments is able to produce enough insulin to process sugars for storage or future use. This protects against diabetic problems in which carbohydrates (sugars and starches) cannot be fully utilized.

**Keeping Your Pancreas Clean.** Avoid refined carbohydrates of any sort. These are processed foods, highly chemicalized, loaded with sugar and salt. These give rise to free radicals that clog your pancreas and block the full production and release of valuable insulin. As sugars and starches are improperly metabolized, end-products or free radicals clog up the bloodstream. This predisposes to more than just diabetes, such disorders as hypoglycemia (blood sugar irregularities), excessive thirst, poor clotting factors, blurred vision, dizziness, lack of energy may also occur. Pamper your pancreas with nourishing foods and avoid those that deposit free radicals in your system.

# NATURAL CARBOHYDRATES CAN GUARD AGAINST FREE RADICALS

To put vigor into your pancreas, select wholesome foods. These include whole grains, especially bran and wheat germ cereals, but they must be natural and without sugar or salt. Fruits and vegetables should be eaten raw unless they absolutely must be cooked. Their high-fiber content is extremely helpful to your pancreas, guarding against the sludgelike formation of free radicals. Select brown rice, whole grain wheat flours or any whole grain flours. With this simple dietary adjustment that calls for saying "no" to any form of sugar or salt, whether from the shaker or in the food you eat, you can invigorate your pancreas and liberate it from the harmful free radicals.

## Increases Insulin, Cleanses Pancreas, Restores Youthful Health

Fluctuating energy levels, excessive thirst, emotional upset made Sarah McG. fearful that her best years were slipping away. Discussing her symptoms with an endocrinologist, she was told to follow a pancreas-pampering program by avoiding sugar and salt, and emphasizing whole foods. Within four days, she had done so well at ridding her pancreas of free radicals, the antioxidant hormones provided her with healthy energy and eradicated her excessive thirst and emotional upset. The increased production of insulin protected her against the threat of diabetes. She looked and felt youthfully alert within eight days! Sarah McG. did it by eating wholesome foods for wholesome health!

**Your Glands Are Powerhouses Of Antioxidants.** With good foods and beverages, you can rid your glands of fragmentary free radicals and let them release their antioxidant hormones, the keys to youth. Hormones are messengers to every nook and cranny of your body; they regenerate your billions of cells to help you achieve and enjoy total youth.

# SUMMARY

1. Unclog your glands so that healthy antioxidant hormones can revitalize your body.
2. Make your adrenals ship-shape with a tasty tonic. It worked wonders for Howard A.J., in washing away aging symptoms, arthritis, and nervousness.
3. Prepare a "Pituitary Power Salad," boost magnesium intake, and enjoy restored vitality. Doris D'A. lost weight and boosted her circulation with a simple program.
4. An invigorated thyroid helps induce total body cellular regeneration. A tasty "Thyroid Tonic" melted Gerald LaM.'s weight, made him calm, cured him of his laziness, and restored youthful vitality in a few days.
5. Sarah McG. followed an easy whole grain, sugar-free, salt-free program to revitalize her pancreas. It helped restore natural insulin release and protect her against diabetes with its complications.

# 14

# Loosen and Liberate Tight Muscles and Enjoy Youthful Flexibility

It happens when you reach for an object on a high shelf. You feel a sudden muscle spasm. You wince with pain. Throbbing pains intensify the gnarled tightness. You have to pause and gasp for breath. When the pain slowly subsides, you are cautious in your range of motion. You will stretch your arms and legs with more extreme caution. You become limited in your movement. As time goes on, your muscles become even more gnarled and twisted. You start to feel helpless, and begin asking others to aid you with tasks that were once very simple.

## BLAME IT ON FREE RADICALS

They become metabolic sediment such as lactic acid. This is a free radical waste product created by normal muscular activity. Ordinarily, these free radicals are washed out through normal eliminative channels (skin pores, respiration, intestines). But if allowed to accumulate, the lactic acid combines with other metabolic fragments and clings to your muscles. These free radicals coat your muscle fibers and "choke" them so that you have a limited range of motion. This can cause "kinks" and "knots" that make you wince or howl with sudden pain when you move your body.

**Free Radicals Invade Muscles.** If allowed to accumulate, these free radicals infiltrate your muscles, cling to your fibers with glue-like stubbornness. Each muscle consists of a bundle of fibers. And each fiber is about the size of a human hair. Penetrating radicals can coat each of these fibers! As this continues, the fibrous muscles become

159

more and more constricted. You develop "tight" muscles, a complaint heard from both older and younger folks. This condition can be controlled with a combination of both antioxidants and body motions. You can uproot the free radicals, break them down, and wash them out of your body. With clean fibrous muscles, you will be able to enjoy youthful flexibility.

## THE ANTIOXIDANT VITAMIN THAT WASHES YOUR MUSCLES

Vitamin D is a dynamic antioxidant because it dispatches calcium throughout your muscular system. This double-barreled action creates biochemical changes within your muscles so that free radicals such as lactic acid are broken up, dissolved, and prepared for speedy elimination. You are rewarded with a full range of free motion.

**Ancients Knew the Value of Sunshine.** During the Greco-Roman era, all praised the value of sunshine as a source of muscular fitness. Athletes and gladiators made use of the sun in training because they saw that it strengthened and enlarged the muscles.

Today, we know that sunshine activates tiny glands within the surface of your skin to manufacture vitamin D. This antioxidant increases the flow of oxygen in your tissues and works with calcium to scour away the free radicals such as lactic acid. This oxygenated activity induces an outpouring of the free radicals through your skin pores. This cleansing process gives your muscles and body a youthfully healthy flexibility.

*Antioxidant Suggestion:* Whenever possible, treat yourself to some sunshine. Keep your head covered and drink adequate liquids to avoid dehydration, especially in warm weather. Just 20 to 30 minutes of sunshine daily will give you a good supply of muscle-washing vitamin D. Calcium is also prompted to perform antioxidant cleansing when influenced by sunshine.

**Vitamin D in Foods.** You may be sensitive to the sun; or else, you may live in an area with inadequate yearly sunshine. You can obtain the antioxidant vitamin D with ordinary foods. These include milk (if the label says vitamin D added), fish liver oils, salmon, tuna, herring, mackerel. Use these foods regularly to nourish your body with important antioxidant vitamin D.

**Foods More Effective Than Sunshine.** Vitamin D is produced by the combined activity of your body oils with the ultraviolet rays of the sun, but the vitamin must be absorbed *through* your skin after it's manufactured *on top* of your skin. It is often washed off before it can be utilized by your body as an antioxidant. Furthermore, if you live in polluted cities or do not get enough sun regularly, you risk having a deficiency. Therefore, foods are a better source of vitamin D. They offer concentrated amounts of vitamin D that work speedily in scraping away free radicals from your muscle fibers.

**Cod Liver Oil: Dynamic Muscle Cleanser.** As a highly concentrated source of vitamin D, along with other important nutrients, cod liver oil works speedily in uprooting, breaking down, and then eliminating metabolic wastes from your muscles. Any fish liver oil is helpful, but cod liver oil appears to be most effective. Available in health food stores, many pharmacies, and supermarkets, try this helpful antioxidant food. If the oily taste turns you off, select mint- or honey-flavored varieties that are available.

*How to Take It:* After breakfast, just one or two tablespoons of fish liver oil gulped down quickly will be adequate for your muscle-cleansing needs. Almost at once the vitamin D helps your metabolic system sweep away lactic acid and other free radicals. This is all you need do. It's simple, but powerfully effective.

**Muscle Cleansing Tonic.** In a glass of any citrus juice (orange, grapefruit, tangerine, or other combinations) add one tablespoon of fish liver oil. Add a half teaspoon of honey. Stir vigorously; better yet, blenderize for just 20 seconds. Drink this tonic once a day, preferably after breakfast.

*Antioxidant Benefits:* Within a half hour, the "Muscle Cleansing Tonic" works at top speed. The ascorbic acid of the citrus juice invigorates the vitamin D of the oil to perform its lactic acid cleansing action. The free radicals are uprooted and eliminated. Muscles start to loosen up; energy is restored; metabolism is improved. You can now do your daily chores, free of back-stabbing pain that was caused by the choking action of the free radicals on your muscle fibers.

## From "Cripple" to "Curvaceous" in Nine Days

As a department store supervisor, Irene E.P. felt stabbing aches whenever she had to reach into a deep bin or up to a high shelf. The muscular pains became worse and worse. Soon she felt crippled. She could scarcely lift her arms above her head to put on a sweater! Irene E.P. felt frightened at the prospect of becoming an invalid. She described her fears to a clinical physiotherapist who advised casting out the free radicals, the encumbering lactic acid wastes from her muscles which were the root cause of her "crippled" feeling. An examination showed that her muscle fibers were coated with this metabolic debris, causing excruciating muscle tightness. Irene E.P. was told to use the "Muscle Cleansing Tonic" just once a day. Within two days she sighed with relief as her limbs became more flexible. By the ninth day, the antioxidant action of vitamin D had so cleansed her muscle fibers, she could enjoy a complete range of motion with nary a twinge of pain. A co-worker said she was now "curvaceous" and no longer "crippled." All this, thanks to the antioxidant action of the "Muscle Cleansing Tonic."

## TWO MINERALS THAT BOOST ANTIOXIDANT REJUVENATION OF "TIRED" MUSCLES

You pick up a spoon; your hand trembles. You try to nap; suddenly your thigh jerks you awake. A nervous twitch makes you edgy all day long. Familiar problems? They could be traced to free radicals that are creating a burden on your muscles. You need antioxidants to cleanse this overlay of waste materials.

**Cleansing Minerals.** There are two minerals that have this dynamic antioxidant action. They help revitalize your muscles, wash away their fatigue, and make you feel alive again. Your weakened muscles now function smoothly. The antioxidants will protect you against sudden jerks, jolts, tremors, tics, twitches, or spasms. To enjoy this muscular control, you need these two antioxidant minerals with cleansing power—*potassium* and *magnesium.*

**Wash Free Radicals from Muscle Pockets.** These two antioxidant minerals cause a unique free radical "washing" reaction right within your muscle pockets. These are the meeting places between your nervous system and muscles, called the neuromuscular junction. At this intersection, electrical impulses pass from your nerves into the muscle where they control its movements. It is precisely in this "muscle pocket" that free radicals will accumulate, much like dust in a corner. If allowed to remain, the free radicals grow thick and become hardened. They block important electrical impulses so your muscles cannot obey the command to move your limb or body in the required direction. This causes muscular cramping and it also predisposes to painful "knots" that leave you crimped up with pain. *Remedy:* Use antioxidants to uproot the blockage of the free radicals and permit a free transfer of messages through your neuromuscular junctions. This is done by intake of the two minerals mentioned previously— magnesium and potassium.

1. *Muscle-Cleansing Magnesium.* This antioxidant scrubs away accumulated free radicals that otherwise block the transfer of messages. Magnesium cleans the delicate muscle fibers and uses its antioxidant ability to relax your muscle so it is not tense. Magnesium will (1) cleanse your muscle, and (2) nourish it to become youthfully flexible. This double-barreled reaction makes magnesium a valuable antioxidant in cleaning your muscle fibers of the restricting free radicals.

2. *Power-Producing Potassium.* This antioxidant balances the conversion of sugar into glycogen, a substance stored in your muscles. Byproducts of incompletely metabolized glycogen gather as free radicals. Stuck in your neuromuscular junction, such molecular fragments create blockages leading to nervous tics, tremors, and spasms. Potassium regulates glycogen storage and prevents its overloading or spilling out which causes rivers of free radicals to clog your muscular system.

You need both magnesium and potassium to balance glycogen levels and cast out constricting free radicals. In so doing, you help loosen and liberate your "tight" muscles and give them more youthful flexibility.

## EASY WAYS TO USE THESE TWO ANTIOXIDANT MINERALS

**Magnesium Food Sources.** Nuts, whole grain breads, cereals, dry beans and peas, dark green vegetables, soy products.

**Potassium Food Sources.** Vegetables (especially the green, leafy variety), oranges, whole grain breads, cereals, sunflower seeds, potatoes (especially the skin), bananas.

*Simple Antioxidant Food Program:* Each day, eat a variety of the aforementioned foods. Strike a balance between raw and cooked foods. Emphasize raw vegetables and fruits, whenever possible, as cooking may deplete some of the nutritional content. You should, however, have cooked beans and peas and potatoes, also, as part of your meal program. They are a vigorous backup vigor to these two antioxidant minerals. And, of course, food supplements are available in potencies specified by your health practitioner.

## Unlocks Muscle Kinks, Unties Painful Knots in Three Days

Getting up from a chair, bending over to tie shoe laces or trying to pick something up from the floor caused Edgar L.L. to howl as he doubled up in pain. At times, it was agony to try and straighten up. Shooting pains went up and down his spinal column, almost "freezing" his back. Even his fingers became stiff at the slightest movement. Edgar L.L. hobbled over to his homeopathic physician who diagnosed the problem as free radical-infested muscles. These molecular fragments clumped together in "pockets," blocking the transfer of impulses. This created a "tieup" which caused spasms and shattering pains during routine motions.

The physician suggested an increase of both magnesium and potassium. Edgar L.L., desperate, made this simple change in his daily diet. Within one day, he could get up and bend over with little pain. By the third day, he was so flexible, he could move his body with the agility of an acrobat. The two antioxidant minerals had washed out the free radicals, unlocked his muscles, and undid the knots. He felt like an athlete, thanks to the antioxidant rejuvenation reaction spurred by these two minerals.

## FUN-TO-DO BODY MOTIONS TO LOOSEN UP TIGHT MUSCLES

Unlock those congested pockets with easy body motions . . . while you sit! These motions speedily improve blood circulation, help wash away free radicals, and free your muscles from blockages.

You can do these exercises at your desk or table. In minutes, they create an antioxidant cleansing of your muscles to help you enjoy more flexible vitality.

**1. Cleansing Neck Muscle Congestion.** Rest hands on table or chair armrests. Keep your shoulders stabilized. Drop your head forward to your chest. Slowly rotate your head to the left, backward, to the right, forward. Repeat three times. Now reverse.

**2. Cleansing Shoulder Muscle Congestion.** Clasp hands behind neck. Keep your head high throughout this motion. Pull in your stomach. Slowly move your elbows back, squeezing your shoulders together. Hold for a slow count of five. Keeping your shoulders squeezed together, unclasp hands and slowly bring arms down sideways. Repeat three times.

**3. Cleansing Chest and Back Congestion.** Sitting, grasp hands on chair armrests. Press downward on hands as if trying to lift yourself off chair. Hold for a slow count of five.

**4. Cleansing Leg Congestion.** Sitting, pull in stomach. Stretch legs forward with feet together and toes pointing upward. Stretch the back muscles of your legs. Hold for a slow count of five.

## CONGESTION-CLEARING MOTIONS
## . . . WHILE YOU STAND

These two simple but amazingly effective antioxidant body motions require standing as they work to dislodge and eliminate free radicals.

**1. Total Body Muscle Cleansing.** Stand erect. Pull in your stomach hard. Keeping your knees straight, transfer your weight to the balls of your feet without raising your heels. Hold for a slow count of five.

**2. Stomach Cleansing.** Stand or walk without raising your chest. Pull in your stomach with maximum effort. Go all the way. Hold for a slow count of five.

*Your Goal:* Follow these body motions every day. Altogether, the six of them take less than 15 minutes. But they do offer hope for freedom from muscular aches and painful spasms because they cleanse away free radicals.

## 20 Minutes Daily Takes 20 Years Off Life

Sagging skin and a general letdown made Pearl O'B. age before her time. She walked with a stooped posture because it was difficult to straighten up. Getting out of bed was an agonizing chore. At times, it was painful for her to hold even the lightest bag of groceries because her muscles twisted up in spasms. Pearl O'B. felt like crying because she was unable to perform simple tasks. The agonizing shooting pains through her tight muscles were too much to bear.

Rather than face the prospect of becoming a bedridden invalid, Pearl O'B. sought help from a local doctor of chiropractic medicine. A thorough diagnostic examination located the cause of her problem. It was muscular overload of free radicals such as lactic acid and metabolic fragmentary wastes. The doctor prescribed 20 minutes daily of the previously mentioned body motions. Pearl O'B. tried them. Within three days she could walk like a youngster, contort her body in all directions, and bounce out of bed. Within two more days she could carry bundles, do household chores and gardening with hardly a pain. By the end of seven days her skin was firm. The body motions, taking just 20 minutes a day, had taken 20 years off her life!

# WHY TOO MUCH SITTING CAN CAUSE INCREASED FREE RADICALS

Sitting is sedentary. It causes great stress on your spine; more so, if you habitually lean forward. Worse, sitting means your muscles become inactive and build up free radicals that may lead to problems such as back pains, especially phlebitis. This condition means inflammation of a vein (usually in the leg) which could be followed by a harmful blood clot, and is symptomatic of free radical congestion. If allowed to remain, the clot can break loose and float up to your lungs, thereby threatening your life.

Free radical congestion caused by prolonged sitting is traced to a pooling of blood in your veins. Since you sit with your knees bent, you constrict the vital veins beneath your knees. This "locks in" free radicals in your veins and the threat of phlebitis emerges. Furthermore, the fragment-burdened muscles cannot control your spinal column. This leads to overall muscular pain.

**Take a Walk and Wash Away Free Radicals.** That's all—walk more and sit less. In so doing, you boost the antioxidant reaction that speeds up your carbohydrate-fat metabolism and facilitates easier removal of these harmful wastes. It's easy to walk more. You could park your car a few blocks from work and walk the rest of the way. Whenever possible, walk up and down several flights of stairs, rather than use the elevator. If you must sit for a long time, plan to get up and walk a few minutes every hour. *Tips:* If possible, elevate your legs while sitting to prevent blood from pooling free radicals in your legs. Always let feet touch the floor when you sit. Do *not* let them hang, since the edge of your seat puts excessive pressure on your thigh veins, choking them, thus causing buildup of molecular litter. So . . . for the sake of your health—take a walk!

# HOW MUSCLE STRETCHING WASHES AWAY TIGHT KNOTS

To increase muscle flexibility, stretch them. To understand how this washes away tight knots, here is a thumbnail description of this antioxidant process.

**Ligaments**—tissues that hold bones together.

**Tendons**—they attach muscles to bones.

Neither of them are flexible or elastic. This means that an exercise that stretches either ligaments or tendons is inadvisable because they do not bounce back. *Tip:* You need to stretch your muscles, instead!

**Why Stretch Muscles?** They are more elastic than ligaments or tendons. Regular muscle stretching gives more flexibility and bounce. Muscles hold your frame together. When healthfully stretched, they loosen and release accumulated free radicals and you have a freer body.

**Stretching Protects Against Muscle Shrinkage.** Prolonged disuse gives rise to a buildup of free radicals that cause blockage and subsequent muscle shrinkage. This puts more pressure on the nerves running through the muscle sheaths, the root cause of aches and pains. *Basic Antioxidant Remedy:* Regular exercise guards against free radical buildup and subsequent shrinkage. Fitness also protects against pain because activity helps wash out free radicals that otherwise could "pinch" your nerves, thus causing discomfort. Follow an exercise program that helps keep you alert, flexible, and youthful.

## SCARF STRETCHING FOR SPEEDY MUSCULAR FLEXIBILITY

All you need is a scarf. That's all. Hold a long scarf in both hands. Slowly try to pull your hands apart. (Keep a tight grip!) Turn to one side, almost bending over while you pull on the scarf. Then slowly stretch and go to your other side. You can also bend forward, even bend backward, while pulling on your scarf. Do this for just five minutes a day.

*Antioxidant Benefit:* The scarf-stretching program unlocks tight pockets of free radicals in your ligaments, tendons, and muscles and helps in their elimination. Once you are free of these wastes, electrical impulses can pass through your muscles, giving them greater flexibility. These antioxidant exercises also help lengthen your muscles and thereby protect against their erosion. The antioxidant exercises guard against muscle knotting so that you can have more flexible muscles. And much of it is done with the use of a scarf!

Free your muscles from pockets of free radicals. Unlock those kinks. Untie those knots. With the use of antioxidant foods and exercises, you can have flexible muscles and youthfulness at any age.

## IN REVIEW

1. Wash away muscular debris with vitamin D.
2. A simple "Muscle Cleansing Tonic" helped Irene E.P. go from "crippled" to "curvaceous" in just nine days.
3. Potassium and magnesium are antioxidant minerals that restore new life to "tired" muscles.
4. Edgar L.L. used two minerals to end his problem of agonizing muscle kinks and painful knots within three days.
5. Follow the fun-to-do and speedily effective body motions (while you sit) that take less than 15 minutes daily to give you a firm and flexible body.
6. Pearl O'B. followed these programs for 20 minutes a day and was rewarded with looking 20 years less than her real age.
7. Sit less. Walk more for greater antioxidant cleansing.
8. Try simple "scarf stretching" to supercharge your body with youthful vitality in minutes.

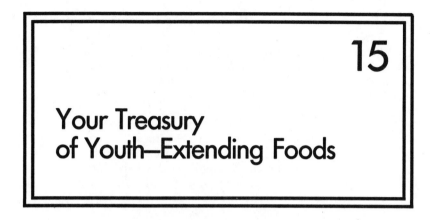

# Your Treasury
# of Youth–Extending Foods

Everyday foods are able to help stimulate your immune system to guard against cellular degeneration and the risk of aging. These tasty foods have specific antioxidants that act as barriers against free radicals; they protect your cells by nourishing the walls and membranes so there is less breakage and deterioration. In so doing, these foods are able to maintain the look and feel of youth in your body. The secret here is that the antioxidants maintain the structure of the tiny organelles and vesicles inside the cells so they can resist viral invaders. They stimulate your cells to produce specific antibodies needed to overcome any threatening microorganisms. These foods act as youth-extenders from within your cells, actively reducing the risk of the rampage of free radicals.

## YOUR EASY YOUTH-EXTENDING PROGRAM

Plan your daily menu around the tasty and versatile foods that will be outlined for you in this chapter. Have a variety of these youth-extenders every day. You will fortify your cells and build youth from within. You will eat your way to cellular revitalization with these everyday, but effective youth-extenders.

### Heals Allergies, Smoothes Skin, Becomes More Flexible

As far back as he could remember, Oscar V. had sinus allergies of one annoying kind after another. Antihistamines, dietary restrictions, and irritating injections offered some relief, but gave him disturbing side effects. His skin became wrinkled. He felt stiff and had tight muscles and a gnarled twisting of his body

169

that made him walk like a stooped invalid. He was getting old far before his time. When he decided to be treated by a holistic physician with emphasis upon cellular nutrition, he was skeptical. But he noticed that when he included as many of the youth-extending foods as possible on his daily menu, he felt better. His immune system resisted allergic reactions so he no longer needed drugs. His skin became smooth again. His arm and leg stiffness changed to flexibility. Oscar V. was no longer a doubter when he could move about with youthful agility and was the picture of glowing youth. He was forever grateful to the holistic physician who said that the real credit should be given to the youth-extending foods for making him look "too young."

## YOUR DIRECTORY OF YOUTH-EXTENDING FOODS

**APPLES.** They contain a natural antioxidant known as *pectin.* This is a natural fat-fighter that limits the amount of potentially destructive fat in your adipose cells. When pectin antioxidants are released in your system, they stimulate your metabolism to scour out your adipose cells, thereby releasing any clusters of free radicals.

**ASPARAGUS.** It has an antioxidant called *asparagine.* This is an alkaloid that will stimulate your metabolism and your kidneys to break down waste deposits. Asparagus also helps in breaking up potentially harmful oxalic acid crystals and protects against cellular deterioration.

**BANANAS.** An excellent source of *potassium, vitamin B6,* and *biotin,* a lesser-known but effective antioxidant B-complex vitamin that is able to nourish your cells and build immunity against the onslaught of harmful free radicals. Bananas help stabilize your blood sugar, improve your heartbeat, and cleanse your neuromuscular network to give you a healthier glow of youth.

**BEETS.** A prime source of a form of low-level *iron* which cleanses your blood cells of free radicals and flushes away waste deposits. Beets also contain natural chlorine, a mineral that energizes your metabolic process and protects against rancid fats by washing them from the cells of your liver, kidneys, and gall bladder.

**BRAN.** An excellent source of non-nutritive fiber or bulk which is able to speed up the transit time of wastes so they do not remain for a dangerously long time in your colon. Many so-called aging illnesses ranging from hemorrhoids, diverticulitis, constipation, diabetes, skin infections, allergies, and gall bladder trouble have been corrected with a boost of bran in the daily diet. It helps to lower cholesterol, a form of fat that can be harmful to your health.

**BREWER'S YEAST.** The dried, pulverized cells of the yeast plant, a strain of *S. cerevisiae,* it is a very powerful composite of most highly concentrated nutrients except for vitamin A, B-12, C, and E. It can be a complete antioxidant food. It is almost 50 percent protein. Brewer's yeast influences your basal metabolism to regenerate your cells and act as a fortress against harmful viral microorganisms.

**CABBAGE.** It possesses a rich content of *iron* and *sulphur* which create antioxidant action by cleansing away fatty deposits and free radicals from your gastrointestinal area. Its mineral combination stimulates your sluggish metabolism to help cast out wastes from infested cells. Enjoy either as raw shredded cabbage in a salad, or cooked, or as a juice.

**CARROTS.** A prime source of valuable *beta-carotene,* predecessor of vitamin A. This antioxidant helps accelerate your metabolism, triggering a waste-flushing reaction. Raw carrot juice is a natural solvent for the free radicals.

**CELERY.** Fresh raw celery has a high concentration of *calcium.* This mineral begins an antioxidant reaction by energizing your endocrine system, producing hormones that help cast out fatty wastes from your cells. Celery is also a prime source of magnesium and iron, two antioxidant minerals that enrich your blood cells and give you youthful immunity.

**CITRUS FRUITS.** These include oranges, grapefruits, tangerines, lemons, and limes. Use them as part of a salad or in the form of juice. Naturally, you do not eat a whole lemon or lime, but you can use a slice in a salad or a cup of tea. These fruits are a prime source of vitamin C, which has an antioxidant action of blocking the accumulation of fatty wastes. Vitamin C will liquefy and dilute the fatty deposits, making it easier to flush them out of your body. Thirst-quenching, citrus fruits are a good source of carbohydrates, those nutrients that give you more energy and a more invigorating metabolism. Whether eaten or taken in juice form, the citrus group is an excellent cell-cleanser.

**CRANBERRIES.** *Malic* and *benzoic acids* are the antioxidant substances found in these red berries that uproot and detoxify the free radicals. Because cranberries are tart, you should use them with a small amount of honey or concentrated fruit juice; or else, add sliced pears or bananas to freshly prepared cranberries. Their juice is a great way to use their powerful antioxidants to stimulate your metabolic system and quench your thirst at the same time. Cranberries are a great and all-natural diuretic.

**CUCUMBER.** This is considered one of the best natural diuretics. It helps release accumulated liquids that might otherwise turn acidic and destroy your cells. The cucumber is a good source of such antioxidants as *silicon* and *sulphur* along with a very high level of *potassium*, thus making it a powerhouse of cell cleansing. You can feel as "cool" as a cucumber and look just as youthful by using this refreshing metabolic stimulant.

**EGGPLANT.** This is an excellent source of *alkaline minerals* that perform an antioxidant reaction by helping to dilute waste accumulations and making them easier to eliminate. You can cook them rapidly in a small amount of boiling water for about five to ten minutes to protect against nutrient loss. They are an excellent source of cleansing roughage that also helps you feel "full" on less food.

**GARLIC.** A prime source of *selenium,* a powerful antioxidant that helps slow the aging process and protects the body against environmental pollution. Selenium in garlic influences your genetic code and guards against the ravages of aging. It especially dissolves the free radicals found in fatty deposits. Selenium works with the vitamin E in garlic to neutralize the free radicals; this protects against damage of not only the cell membranes, but other vital materials in your body, especially your genetic materials. Garlic is a rich concentration of antioxidants that stabilize your blood pressure, enrich your bloodstream, boost your powers of immunity, and give you stamina and youthful vitality. Use garlic either raw or cooked to benefit from its protective qualities.

**NUTS.** These are dry stone fruits, a prime source of meatless *protein*. A rich concentration of many nutrients, these foods introduce the antioxidant *zinc* which is needed to build collagen (of which the membranous cell walls are made), to keep out viral invaders. But don't go nutty with nuts! Although a plentiful source of zinc notwithstanding, you are also munching on many calories. A handful will go a long way.

**OILS, VEGETABLE.** They assist in the breakdown and synthesis of accumulated fat in your adipose cells. They provide antioxidants to act as insulators in maintaining body temperature. They also protect your essential organs (heart, liver, and kidneys) and form essential constituents of cell membranes by regulating the intake and removal of wastes and transporting essential nutrients. In particular, vegetable oils have *linoleic acids,* nutritional antioxidants that are needed to break down fatty accumulations. Just two or three tablespoons of your favorite vegetable oil in your salad daily may well be all you need to keep up your antioxidant levels.

**ONIONS.** Onions have antioxidants that are able to slow down platelet aggregation, which can otherwise lead to serious blood clots. Onions are also prime sources of antioxidants that are able to keep your cholesterol level in check and inhibit misshapen cellular growths that could be a threat to your life.

**PARSLEY.** Very rich in nutrients, this vegetable is able to stimulate your metabolism. It has antioxidant properties which boost oxygen metabolism and rejuvenate the action of your thyroid and adrenal glands to help wash out free radicals. The antioxidant elements in parsley are proportioned in such a manner that they help maintain the elasticity and youthfulness of your blood vessels, particularly your capillaries and arterioles.

**PEPPERS.** A little-known but excellent source of *ascorbic acid* (vitamin C) which is a key in building collagen, the walls of your membranes. One average green pepper contains twice the amount of vitamin C as an orange. When peppers "age," they turn red and fill up with an excellent supply of vitamin A, a truly miraculous antioxidant. Enjoy peppers, green or red, and you may well enjoy healthy cells and youthfulness, too.

**SEEDS.** A "must" in your youth-extending program, sunflower, sesame, pumpkin, and squash, seeds are rich sources of *zinc* (a dynamic antioxidant) and *protein*. Seeds also contain an antioxidant considered as a "protease inhibitor" which seems to protect against cancerous cellular growths. Plan to use seeds on a daily basis. Just a handful will help provide a good amount of antioxidants that will keep harmful damage to your cells at a minimum.

**SOYBEANS.** They contain an antioxidant substance called *lecithin* which releases a byproduct known as *lecithin cholesterol acyltransferase* (LCAT). This byproduct serves as a barrier and defense mechanism against viral microorganisms that would otherwise threaten your molecules. As free radicals are broken down by LCAT, they can be more easily flushed out of your system. It is the LCAT antioxidant process, via eating soybeans, that helps guard against molecular breakdown and premature aging.

**SPROUTS.** More than just grassy accoutrement to a sandwich or salad, sprouts have extremely high levels of many nutrients, especially *vitamin C*. Mung bean sprouts are especially high in *calcium* and *magne-*

*sium* which are vital for helping the metabolic process. Wheat sprouts block the genetic damage to cells caused by some free radicals. In any combination, a large serving of sprouts (preferably raw) will help bolster your defense mechanisms against the aging process.

SWEET POTATOES. Botanically, they have no relation to the white potato and belong in a class by themselves. Their gold-colored flesh is a prime source of *beta-carotene,* the valuable antioxidant that fight erosion in your cells. As a healthful accompaniment to a main course or as a "snack" by itself, the sweet potato is a "must" in your quest for youth foods.

TOMATOES. Rich in *vitamin C* and natural *citric acids* that help stimulate your metabolic and immune processes, the tomato and its juice act as a diuretic by stimulating your kidneys to wash out the clinging free radicals. With the use of enzyme-activated minerals, the tomato signals your kidneys to cleanse your system of its accumulated viral microorganisms that pose a threat to your health.

WATERMELON. This is a prime source of minerals that appear to rejuvenate your system and boost the washing out of wastes. If you feel "overloaded" or "clogged up" and are unable to rid yourself of radical fragments, then several slices of watermelon should help do the fat-washing trick.

WHEAT GERM. An excellent source of B-complex vitamins, especially *thiamine,* which energizes your metabolic system. It also contains *vitamin E,* which protects the fat-containing body tissues from damaging reactions from rancid oxygen. A one-ounce serving of wheat germ provides 62 percent of polyunsaturated oil, which is vital in dislodging free radicals and keeping your cells free of impediment.

YOGURT. This is fermented milk that is rich in calcium. It is easier to digest for those who are intolerant to ordinary milk. It has a fine curd which speeds up assimilation at a faster rate. Yogurt contains *lactobacillus* bacteria, which has an antioxidant action of destroying harmful microorganisms and establishing a good environment for better digestive ability. A cup or two of yogurt daily (be sure it has no sugar or salt; read labels), will create gastrointestinal vigor that is the foundation of super youth!

The preceding foods are available in almost all health food stores as well as your neighborhood supermarket or produce dealer. Make them a part of your shopping list to give you molecular rejuvenation and help you live longer and better.

## "Fountain of Youth is on My Kitchen Table"

The so-called bloom of youth faded as Kay MacL. became pale, walked with a stooped gait, was so slow with her reflexes that she was afraid to cross busy thoroughfares by herself. She developed the "shakes," which made it difficult for her to button her clothes. Kay MacL. was afraid to lose her dressmaking position because she felt herself becoming feeble. She was hardly in her fiftieth year! She refused to believe her condition was hereditary just because her parents had aged early. She was told by a nutritionist that with the knowledge about antioxidants, the modern person could use foods as antidotes against molecular disintegration, a prime cause of aging. Her parents did not know of this scientific breakthrough. But the nutritionist made this discovery available to Kay MacL. by providing her with a list of the preceding youth foods. They were to be part of her daily diet along with other foods, of course. Kay MacL. was amazed at how they worked so swiftly. Her skin firmed up and had the familiar bloom of roses. She could walk with vitality and her hand was steady. She could work overtime with great energy, more so than her younger co-dressmakers. When asked for her secret of rejuvenation, she told them it came from nature's horn of plenty, and that the "fountain of youth is on my kitchen table!"

How can you preserve your youth? How can you reverse the tide of aging and enjoy restoration of your youth? The answer is with youth-extending foods that are concentrated sources of antioxidants that can rebuild your millions of molecules so that you can resist the threat of their disintegration and prolong your prime of life. These youth-extending foods can help make you immune to aging. And they can begin their rejuvenation at once. So can you!

## SUMMARY

1. Plan your easy youth-extending program with the assortment of tasty and easily obtainable foods. They are prime sources of the secret of rejuvenation; namely, antioxidants that rebuild your molecular network and put you on the road to youth.

2. Oscar V. used these antioxidant foods to correct allergies, smooth out his skin, and regain flexibility in his arms and legs.
3. Kay MacL. was saved from premature aging with the use of these antioxidant foods. She would tell others only that the "fountain of youth is on my kitchen table."

# 16

# Rejuvenation Secrets from Europe and the Orient

Visitors to other continents are amazed at the youthful appearance of so many of their natives. Europeans and Orientals, in particular, have younger-looking skin, show much more energy, and are amazingly free of many of the so-called illnesses of old age as in North America. How do these people remain healthfully and vigorously young in their sixth, seventh, and eighth decades of life?

The answer is partly traditional, whereby they use folk remedies, special foods, and simple home programs that they know will control aging. Better yet, many of these rejuvenation secrets help halt and then reverse the aging clock. In particular, these secrets are able to block infections by forming antibodies, the immunological proteins that chemically fight off the invading microorganisms that would cause physical and emotional aging. Researchers have delved into these secrets and applied them to modern usage in the United States. They have noted that you can feel and look healthier, younger, and more beautiful with these rejuvenation programs that you can follow right at home.

Here is a collection of these so-called folk remedies that have scientific merit in that they are able to protect against the harmful ravages of free radicals and prolong the prime of your life. Most of them work almost immediately, so begin watching for the rejuvenation process right away!

## YOUTH SECRETS FROM SWEDEN

The glowing skin and the effervescence so typical of people from Sweden may well be traced to these traditional youth programs.

**Rose Hips for Cellular Rejuvenation.** These are the small, cherry-sized, fully ripened, orange-red fruits just below the rose flowers. Certain varieties of rose bushes produce this top-notch fruit, such as the *rosa villosa, rosa canina,* and *rosa rugosa.* A traditional Swedish diet calls for using rose hips either as a jam, as a powder to be mixed with fruit juices, or as a sugar substitute. It is a richly concentrated source of vitamin C, the antioxidant that builds collagen, the substance that provides stability and tensile strength for all body tissues. Prepare a rejuvenating tonic simply by mixing a tablespoon of rose hips powder with any citrus juice. The bioflavonoids in the citrus juice act as synergists with the vitamin C in rose hips to make a biologically potent youth beverage. Drink just one or two glasses daily and see the results immediately. It is an old Swedish custom and it has proven its value in the glowing faces of its natives. Rose hips are available at health food stores everywhere.

**Whey is the Way to Colonic Rejuvenation.** Whey is the liquid left over when cheese is made from milk. When milk coagulates, the solid part, or curds, is removed and the remaining liquid is called whey. In Sweden, whey is traditionally dehydrated and used on a daily basis. Whey is close to 80 percent pure lactose, the substance that nourishes the important acidophilus bacteria in your colonic region. Whey is able to protect against the growth of harmful microorganisms there. It is traditionally believed that auto-toxemia (self-poisoning) through proliferation of metabolic free radicals in the large intestine is one of the main causes of aging. The natural antidote is to use whey to keep the colon in a state of clean rejuvenation. It is the key to correction of constipation, which also is an aging symptom. In the United States, whey is available as a powder or tablet in many health food stores, as well as special diet food outlets. Just mix the powder with some fruit or vegetable juice and drink two glasses daily. It is a natural miracle food that helps you enjoy a longer lifespan.

**Facial Sauna at Home.** Cleanse your face of blemishes with the use of this simple traditional Swedish technique. Put two tablespoons of your favorite herbs (natives of Sweden use pine needles or birch leaves, which may be available locally at herbal outlets) in a pot of water. Bring it to a boil. Remove pot and put on a metal or wooden base to avoid burning of the surface. Cover your head with a big bath towel. Lower your head over the pot and steam your face for up to 10 minutes. Keep turning your face so that all areas, including the neck, are treated to this aromatic facial cleanser evenly. The herbal steam will open pores, cleanse out wastes, and create an antioxidant purification through the action of the herbs so that you will emerge looking youthfully clean.

## YOUTH SECRETS FROM FINLAND

Steam heat and water form the antioxidant rejuvenation secrets for the people of this hardy country.

**Saunas Chase Out Free Radicals.** Known as a Finnish steambath, a sauna produces a moist steamy heat that will open up your pores so that harmful free radicals can be washed out of your system. The secret here is that the comfortably high heat creates an artificially induced fever that combats the growth of viruses and stimulates your glands to build a defensive line against hostile invaders. Ask your health practitioner if a Finnish-style sauna is suitable for your particular condition. Just 20 to 30 minutes in a sauna, once or twice a week, can help cleanse your body and control the level of free radicals.

**Finnish Cleansing Bath.** To begin, do not eat for two hours before using this method. If you have any kind of cardiovascular illness, ask your doctor about the advisability of using this very warm cleansing bath. *How to Do It:* Fill a tub with water at about 98°. Remain *under* the water with only your head sticking out. Let hot water run slowly from the tap so that the temperature of the water increases a few more degrees, up to about 102°F. Just soak for a half hour. Your body temperature should equal that of the water if you remain totally immersed. Then climb out, wrap yourself in a thick Turkish towel, climb into bed and cover yourself with a warm blanket. Remain in bed for an hour or more so that your temperature slowly returns to normal. You will be sweating all this time. This is a natural fever that will wash out the harmful free radicals and enable antioxidants to repair and rebuild your body.

**Rye Is a Youth Food in Finland.** For these hardy people, whole rye is considered the secret of life itself. Reason? It contains the *germ*, the reproductive power that promotes perpetuation of the species. In particular, the Finns like sourdough rye bread (available locally in many health food stores or specialty bake shops) because it has lactic acid which makes the grains more easily available for assimilation. It is this lactic acid that acts like an antioxidant in protecting against formation of harmful free radicals. And it is available in sourdough rye bread and also in whole rye bread and cereal products. It is the tasty way to help keep yourself youthfully healthy.

# YOUTH SECRETS FROM RUMANIA

This country is well known for its Gerovital rejuvenation therapy, also known as novocaine or procaine, or popularly dubbed KH-3 by the famous Dr. Ana Aslan. It is not permitted to be sold in the United States because it needs to undergo stringent tests by the Food and Drug Administration. But there are alternatives that use the same novocaine principle, but with natural foods.

**Youth Elixir with Procaine Power.** The use of bioflavonoids, concentrated segments found near the rind of citrus fruits, together with rose hips powder and one teaspoon of wheat germ oil will give you a comparable invigoration as with the famous Gerovital. Just blenderize segments of any citrus fruits (including the white, stringy portions) with some rose hips powder and the oil. You will get a powerful combination of antioxidants that provide a feeling of total well-being. Known as a "Youth Elixir," it works by producing a combination formula that improves cellular metabolism and glandular functions in a biological manner.

**Cucumber Beauty Cream.** Throughout Rumania, the cucumber is a basic staple. It is a prime source of many minerals, especially selenium, which you know is one of the most potent antioxidants available. Rumanian women look refreshingly young because of their daily use of the cucumber eaten as part of a salad. But one secret is using the cucumber as a skin rejuvenator. *How to Make It:* Slice a cucumber into one-inch pieces. Place in a blender together with ¼ cup milk, ½ teaspoon honey, one teaspoon crushed ice. Blenderize only until mixture has the consistency of porridge (about three seconds at low speed). Now use as a mask over your face, throat, hands, and anywhere else that needs softening. Rest for 30 minutes. Let the antioxidants soak into your skin and cast out the free radicals. Then splash off with tepid and cold water. *Suggestion:* Use this "Cucumber Beauty Cream" at least once a day. Within a few days, the antioxidant rejuvenation reactions will be happily observed as wrinkles smooth out, color is restored, blemishes are gone, and you look years younger.

## Brightens Up Skin, Rolls Back Years in Seven Days

Janet M. was bothered by advancing age in the form of sallow skin, with unsightly blotches and wrinkles. She kept using heavier and heavier makeup to disguise the unsightly truth. Her cosmetician sympathized and said that with the use of Rumanian youth secrets she could correct the cause of her aging skin; namely, the wastes in her cells. She suggested that Janet M. try the Youth Elixir and also the "Cucumber Beauty Cream." Desperate, she began the programs. She enjoyed the elixir and did feel refreshed from the beauty cream. But she was soon exhilarated when she saw her skin smoothing out, her wrinkles vanishing, her blotches fading away. She began to experience unbelievable energy as the antioxidants restored and restructured her molecular framework. Janet M. was forever grateful to the cosmetician for these secrets. Within seven days, she felt (and looked) as if she had rolled back the years!

# YOUTH SECRETS FROM FRANCE

Long known for having exquisitely attractive women and vibrant men, France may well be considered years ahead of other western countries in recognizing the importance of rebuilding youth from within. Some of their secrets can show results for you almost from the start.

**Cabbage for Internal Youth.** This vegetable is a major staple among the youth-seeking French, and for good reason. It is an excellent source of the two basic antioxidants, vitamin C and selenium. When cabbage is eaten either raw (as part of a salad) or cooked, it provides a rich concentration of both of these valuable youth-builders. Also, many French people have found that a glass of freshly squeezed cabbage juice, flavored with a bit of lemon juice and a pinch of your favorite herbal spice, does provide a feeling of exhilaration. The juice is a rich source of antioxidants and is looked upon as a "youth tonic" by the forever young French.

**Garlic Is a Powerful Antioxidant.** It is rare to be served a dish of food in France without the ingredient, garlic. The French look upon garlic as a "fountain of youth." It releases selenium, along with specific anti-bacterial properties that engulf the potentially harmful free radicals and deactivate them so that your molecules remain immune to such dangers. Garlic is a "must" in French cooking. Even bread is treated to a taste of garlic because a little bit goes a long way. The amazing stamina and eternal youth of the garlic-loving French attributes to the power of this vital antioxidant food.

**Onions Are Natural Antioxidants.** Famed for using onions in just about every recipe, let alone the well-known French onion soup, the French know this vegetable has antioxidants that protect blood platelets from clinging together. The substances in onions help dislodge festering free radicals and get them out of your body. Onions are dynamic molecule cleansers and the French always praise them for keeping up their *joie de vivre*.

## YOUTH SECRETS FROM ITALY

From this Mediterranean land, the radiant joy and robust health of the people can be largely attributed to their desire to use specific foods. These certain foods help them live longer and better.

**Cold-Pressed Oils Offer Warm Life.** Taken from any variety of grains, cold-pressed oils offer the Italians a supply of vitamin E as well as polyunsaturated fatty acids that are needed to boost antioxidant power to help give them youthful immunity to many illnesses, including that of old age! The use of cold-pressed oils can be seen in their smooth and well moisturized skin. Cold-pressed oils are a means of dissolving free radicals beneath the skin surface, moisturizing the cells, and thereby plumping up your body envelope, your skin. Use cold-pressed oils whenever possible and give yourself a younger body.

**Sources of Rejuvenating Oils.** With the cold-pressed method, the oil is expelled from various seeds by mechanical pressure without the use of chemicals. A variety of such oils include those from the almond, apricot, corn, garlic, olive, peanut, rice, safflower, sesame, soy, walnut, and wheat germ, to name a few sources. Your health food store or supermarket should have a selection of these oils to suit your palate and body. Use them for your salad dressings, marinating, baking, and in just about any recipe instead of hydrogenated or hardened fats such as lard or animal fats.

## Corrects Stiff Limbs, Smooths Skin, Improves Hair

Dolores N.I. was troubled by increasing stiffness of her limbs. She began showing deep wrinkles and unsightly dandruff appeared on her thinning hair. Was she getting old? She was hardly in her early fifties. On a vacation cruise, she asked the Italian hostess how she was so young-looking. She was told the secret which called for three to four tablespoons of cold-pressed oils daily, either as part of a salad or mixed with a vegetable juice. Dolores N.I. tried the simple program. In three days, she had more flexible agility, a smoother skin and with hardly any wrinkles, and was most delighted by having conquered the dandruff problem and growing thicker hair! Dolores N.I. had allowed antioxidants in the oil to cleanse away impediments and granular free radicals that were causing premature aging. She admitted her age to the hostess and was astonished to hear that the hostess was much older than Dolores was. She was told, "Just keep using the oil and you'll look younger than me!"

**Fresh, Green, Leafy Vegetables.** In these we find valuable minerals, especially selenium, which can reverse the aging process in a short time. Italians are known for their fabulous salads using garlic, onions, and oils, all of which are high in antioxidants. Plan to eat fresh raw vegetable salads every day and you will soon see the beneficial results.

## YOUTH SECRETS FROM SWITZERLAND

Nestled between high mountains, this tiny country boasts one of the highest ratings of health and longevity. They have discovered a few simple but potent secrets of extending the prime of life.

**Whole Grains in the Morning.** Some of the leading Swiss health spas have a rule that a breakfast of raw whole grains is a "must" for your survival. These grains are excellent sources of polyunsaturated fatty acids, as well as vitamin E and many minerals that act as a buffer against the threat of invading free molecules. The Swiss know that a good whole grain breakfast is a powerful way to build immunity to many ailments, including so-called old age. You can follow the program with any raw whole grain breakfast. Use no sugar; no salt. Fresh fruit slices are good and provide needed vitamin C. For a liquid, try yogurt, milk, or fruit juice.

**Begin with a Vegetable Salad . . . End with a Fruit Salad.** The Swiss aging specialists have long recognized that a raw vegetable salad boosts digestive enzymes to prepare your system for the food that follows. This corrects any problems of poor metabolism and assures better assimilation of nutrients. Eat a raw vegetable salad at the start of a meal. End with raw fruits to produce better digestion and enzymatic breakdown of food so that important nutrients can be assimilated. This simple two-step eating program may well be the most important secret of youth from the mountainous country of ageless Switzerland.

# YOUTH SECRETS FROM BULGARIA

Considered the longest-living people of Europe, the Bulgarians use simple, but amazingly effective, food programs to help nourish their bodies and protect themselves against premature aging.

**Yogurt for Youth.** It is well known that Bulgarians consume more soured milk in the form of yogurt than any other people in the world. It is believed that fermented or soured milk products help prevent putrefication in the colon and guard against auto-toxemia which is the key to living longer and better. Bulgarians are the tallest and healthiest people of Europe. They have more centenarians (people who live beyond the 100 age mark) than any other civilized nation. Yogurt as a youth-restoring food may well be the reason, and it is worth a tasty test.

**Sauerkraut Can Control Free Radicals.** The Bulgarians have traditionally looked to sauerkraut as a healing food. Made of raw cabbage which is then fermented, it provides valuable minerals and the potent antioxidant, selenium. Whether store-bought or homemade, it should be salt-free so it can work freely to build strong molecular structure and good levels of immunity.

# YOUTH SECRETS FROM SOVIET RUSSIA

From behind the iron curtain there are reports of people living more than just to the century mark, but even beyond. What are the secrets of this incredible longevity? Some of them include:

**Bee Pollen.** This is believed to contain all of the known nutrients in microscopic amounts but in a nature-created balance. Many Russian scientists have found that beekeepers and others who eat bee pollen regularly are able to avoid premature aging and its accompanying infirmities. Pollen contains *deoxiribosides* and *sterines,* plus a *gonadotropic plant hormone* to stimulate your reproductive glands. These are antioxidant factors that increase your immunological mechanisms and stimulate rejuvenating activity from within. Bee pollen is available in tablet, capsule, or granule form at most local health food stores.

**Buckwheat is a Youth Food.** It has been reported that Russians who eat buckwheat regularly have more resistance to high blood pressure and cardiovascular ailments. The reason? Buckwheat contains *rutin,* a bioflavonoid that acts as an antioxidant in helping to reduce pressure and soothe the circulatory system. Buckwheat proteins are of high quality and help your billions of cells to resist bacterial invasion. Use buckwheat as a nutritious cereal and in baking and eat your way to youth.

# YOUTH SECRETS FROM THE ORIENT

From the East, we see that the long-living Orientals have used several foods as staples for thousands of years. The amazing capacity for work and activity that Orientals have may well be traced to the antioxidant powers of these foods.

**Millet Can Be a Miracle Food.** A complete protein food millet contains all essential amino acids and is comparable in biological value to meat. An alkaline food, it guards against acid formation and cellular disintegration. Furthermore, millet alkalines help dissolve free radicals and counteract harmful microorganism invasion. You can enjoy millet cereal that tastes similar to oatmeal. Millet is available at many health food stores, gourmet food shops, and some supermarkets.

**Sesame Seeds: Open the Doorway to Youth.** Sesame seeds are especially good sources of the amino acid, *methionine*, and are rich in *lecithin*, an effective antioxidant that keeps your blood vessels cleansed of free radicals. When mashed and combined with chick peas or garbanzos, this paste is called *tahini*. A bit of honey added to sesame seeds will make *halvah*. Both are tasty ways to nourish your glands and open the doorway to new youth.

Tap the wellsprings of youth that gush forth in Europe and the Orient and give your body an ample supply of antioxidants that help you live longer, younger, and healthier.

## MOST IMPORTANT

1. Sweden offers youth foods that work wonders in a short time.
2. Become as hardy and youthful as people in Finland with their home programs.
3. Rumania offers several youth secrets that are powerhouses of antioxidants.
4. Janet M. used the "Youth Elixir" and "Cucumber Beauty Cream" to brighten her skin and roll back the years. She saw results in seven days.
5. Vive la France with their beauty and youth secrets you can now use for swift results.
6. Dolores N.I. used a youth secret from Italy to correct stiffening limbs and improve her skin and hair.
7. Switzerland, Bulgaria, and Soviet Russia, together with the Orient offer a cornucopia of youth secrets that work immediately.

# 17

## Your Antioxidant Lifetime Guide To Help You Stay Forever Young

You can live a long time without getting old if you use antioxidants as part of your program for staying young, healthy, and active. With the use of these cell builders, you can help build resistance to the basic cause of aging—cellular deterioration. It is *not* the passage of time that brings on so-called aging. Instead, it is the destruction of your cells by the damaging free radicals that shortens your lifespan.

## WHY DOES AGING HAPPEN?

A free radical, which is a fragment of a molecule that has been torn away from its source during a "deleterious reaction" joins another molecule. It can do this because it has an unpaired electron which gives it the power to damage the molecule it attempts to join. This can cause a chain reaction of molecular disintegration.

This happens because oxidation in your bloodstream forms these free radicals. Even in small amounts, they cause aging. They cause their damage by reacting with DNA–RNA, the blueprints by which your cells are replicated. But when bombarded by free radicals, these blueprints lose their ability to decode some of the instructions given by your biological system. A cumulative effect of the damage done by free radicals formed by oxidation can cause aging. If there were no crossed wires, the DNA–RNA process would work well, bring about the replication of new cells, and youth could continue forever. But the presence of free radicals causes the process to go awry, and the cells become incomplete, inactive, and become unable to properly duplicate themselves. You can see this in the form of aging.

In brief, aging reflects a weakness of the immune system because of the cellular breakdown caused by the free radicals. Therefore, by selectively changing the immune system through the means of better nutrition and better living methods, it may well be possible to put the DNA–RNA back on an even keel. This could very well help protect against such age-causing problems as cardiovascular disorders, stroke, respiratory problems, glandular weakness, atherosclerosis, and emotional depression, to name just a few symptoms of aging.

## HOW ANTIOXIDANTS HOLD THE KEY TO PERPETUAL YOUTH

Must you just sit there and let the free radicals make you old before your time? Definitely not, with the availability of antioxidants, considered to be a major breakthrough in the search for perpetual youth.

Antioxidants are substances that defuse the power of the free radicals. *Example:* Free radicals are oxygen molecules that are highly unstable and react in the body to cause degenerating changes. But antioxidants change free radicals into stable oxygen and block their efforts of attacking cells. Furthermore, an abundance of antioxidants will devour and wash out free radicals and prevent their formation, protect your cells, and give you effective immunity in resisting illnesses. By protecting aerobic organisms, these youth extenders are able to guard against oxidation/reduction reactions in your cells. Within this fascinating web of science, we see that we are on the threshold of discovering the key to perpetual youth.

## HOW TO USE ANTIOXIDANTS FOR A YOUTHFUL LIFE

They are found not only in foods, but in a more healthful lifestyle. You need to improve your lifestyle to enjoy a prolonged lifespan. Here is a set of programs that can restructure your biological molecular foundation to help free you of oxygen rancidity, the real cause of aging.

**VITAMIN E.** It helps lower cholesterol levels, boosts your immune system, reduces the incidence of cellular overload. It protects against toxins and poisons, both those encountered from the atmosphere, as well as from food additives, or those your own body manufactures from a poor diet, incomplete digestion and elimination, and too little exercise. *Sources:* wheat germ oil, eggs, leafy green vegetables, fish, cold-pressed vegetable oils.

**SELENIUM.** This mineral appears to preserve tissue elasticity by delaying oxidation of polyunsaturated fatty acids which could cause solidification of tissue proteins. It neutralizes the free radicals and protects your cell membranes and other vital organs and glands. Selenium also offers some protection against cigarette smoke. It is believed to protect against such environmental oxidants as heavy metals (cadmium, lead, mercury), certain organic compounds (halogenated hydrocarbons), alcoholic drinks, and the ozone and nitrogen dioxide of air pollution. *Sources:* Lean meats and seafoods are the best sources. Eggs and dairy products are adequate. Grains, depending on the soils where they were grown, can supply modest amounts.

**VITAMIN C.** It stimulates the immune system, blocks formation of blood clots, protects you against strokes and degenerative heart diseases. It is vital to collagen formation, the connective substance in all body cells. It also fights the toxic effects of smoke and pollution. Vitamin C helps in healing and in production of red blood cells. *Sources:* fresh citrus fruits and their juices, green peppers, vegetables.

**CYSTEINE.** An amino acid that is directly concerned with stimulating the immune system. Be sure to double-check the spelling of any product purchased because it is *cysteine* and not *systine* (the oxidized form of cysteine) that stimulates the system. *Sources:* Most animal products have this but you would need to consume a large amount for cysteine to help knock out the threat of free radicals, so supplements are available. Discuss potency with your health practitioner.

**VITAMIN A or BETA-CAROTENE.** It is needed to increase the size of your thymus (the fist-sized lymph gland behind your breastbone) to produce the vigorous T-lymphocytes. These cells are considered your first line of defense against deterioration. Vitamin A produces antibodies that combat invading microorganisms. If you prefer meatless sources, beta-carotene is the yellow pigment in fruits and vegetables that is transformed into vitamin A. In either form, it is a "must" for the anti-aging program. *Sources:* fish liver oils, dairy products, liver, meats, eggs, seafood. Beta-carotene is also found in carrots, cantaloupe, peaches, squash, tomatoes, green and yellow fruits and vegetables.

## Five Antioxidants Reverse Tide of Aging

He was in his early sixties, yet Morton DeP. looked and acted much, much older. His memory was drifting. He tired easily when walking around the block. He developed an arthritic-like stiffness that reduced his ability to use his hands. He was often confined to a wheelchair because his legs would give out. He looked haggard and the slightest breeze made him cough and sneeze and feel chilly in any climate. He might have been confined to an "old age" home had it not been for the help of a nutritionally educated gerontologist (specialist in older-aged patients). His problem was diagnosed as a deficiency in antioxidants. Morton DeP. was given a diet featuring the five all-important antioxidants: vitamin E, selenium, vitamin C, cysteine, vitamin A or beta-carotene. Results? It took three weeks to help undo the damage caused by the rampaging free radicals, but by the end of the third week Morton DeP. had a sharp memory. He had so much energy, he could walk up and down four flights of stairs with the greatest of ease. His face looked healthy and alert. He no longer was sensitive to the climate. On a cool evening, he did not even need a sweater. He was warm and young, thanks to the antioxidant program. These youth extenders had done just that . . . prolonged and restored his prime of life!

# ANTIOXIDANT PROGRAMS TO HELP YOU ENJOY FREEDOM FROM AGING

Nutritional antioxidants are the foundation upon which you should plan your lifetime guide to perpetual youth. Health-building antioxidants include a variety of different programs in daily living. Follow them on a day-to-day basis and watch yourself feel younger in a short time. You will then see how these antioxidant reactions hold the key to rejuvenation.

**Keep Yourself Physically Active.** Regular exercise gives a vital antioxidant benefit. Aerobic exercise (jogging, running, cycling, swift walking, stair climbing, and swimming) will help your muscles draw fat from your blood for metabolic needs which keeps body fat in check. A program of regular exercise is a must for antioxidant rewards.

**Take an Hour Walk Every Day.** Perhaps more, if conditions allow. Walking causes an increased blood supply which will keep your tissues warm. In the same way that a fever helps to kill viruses, warm bodies are more likely to ward them off. This is the reason vigorously active people have fewer infections and recover from illnesses more quickly. Walking for an hour or more every day will give you this antioxidant boost in the form of warmth and also greater immunity.

**Protect Yourself Against Stress.** It is a potent toxin and can be as destructive as chemical pollution in your system. It wears away your molecules. It is involved in hypertension, cardiovascular disease, and mental breakdown. You need to assess your particular stress levels. Know how much can you take. Match this with your individual needs, ambitions, and performance. Everyone has a pace at which they work best. Find yours. Know your limits. Do not exceed them. Develop a positive mental attitude so you can cope with the responsibilities of the day.

**Have a Daily Rest Period.** This means a period of complete relaxation and escape from mental and physical tension. It is helpful when you are able to lie down in a quiet place. Allow your stiff, tense muscles to go limp one after the other while your eyes are closed. Breathe slowly but rhythmically. Ten minutes can refresh you as much as two hours of sleep. Begin by relaxing your feet and continue upward with your legs, thighs, stomach, chest, shoulders, arms and neck. Develop regular rest periods and the antioxidant effect of being refreshed will go a long way toward helping you live longer, better, and younger.

**Sleep Is Important.** It is an antioxidant in that it helps repair the stresses of the day. During restful sleep, heart rate and breathing slow down considerably and your body temperature drops. At the same time, your muscles and blood vessel walls relax, thus reducing your blood pressure. Your hard-working organs enjoy rest and revitalization. While each person's needs are different, an average of eight to ten hours of sleep should be your goal. How can you tell if you are getting enough sleep? When you wake up feeling refreshed!

**Control Your Weight.** Obesity is contrary to antioxidant healing. Excess weight can cause an excess of free radicals that will create serious problems in your cells and tissues. By keeping your weight within your proper limit, you will have better circulation and more effective antioxidant function.

**Drink Lots of Water.** Your body is like a system of rubber tubes which hold about ten gallons of water. Six to eight glasses of water are needed to replenish this system every day. Water helps dissolve the free radicals and carry them out of your body. Drink water before or after meals, but not during a meal, and never to "wash foods down." You should not dilute the antioxidants in foods by drinking excessive amounts of water while eating. Instead, chew food carefully and thoroughly and swallow without gushes of water following.

**Emphasize Whole Foods.** Simply stated, these are foods as created by nature and neither refined nor fragmented. Wherever possible, have whole grain breakfast cereals, cold-pressed oils, freshly prepared fruit and vegetable juices. lean meats, and all the other foods that come from as natural a source as possible since they are prime sources of valuable antioxidants.

With these guidelines, you will be able to do more than postpone old age, but you can prevent it with the help of building inner immunity against molecular injury. You can give yourself a new lease on life with this knowledge of extended youth. Prepare yourself for a new era of buoyant health and total freedom from aging. Live longer, live younger with the amazing power of antioxidants. Begin today and become younger tomorrow!

# SUMMARY

1. With the use of an antioxidant way of life, you can restructure and regenerate your molecules to give you a longer and disease-free lifestyle.
2. Morton DeP. used five basic everyday antioxidants to reverse the tide of aging.
3. Refer to the collection of better health living programs in this book and build them into your day-to-day routine and discover the youth-restoring rewards in a short time.

# Index